The Prostate
Cancer Sourcebook

The Prostate Cancer Sourcebook

How to Make Informed Treatment Choices

Marcus H. Loo, M.D.,
and Marian Betancourt

John Wiley & Sons, Inc.

New York • Chichester • Weinheim • Brisbane • Singapore • Toronto

The information contained in this book is not intended to serve as a replacement for professional medical advice. Any use of the information in this book is at the reader's discretion. The author and publisher specifically disclaim any and all liability arising directly or indirectly from the use or application of any information contained in this book. A health care professional should be consulted regarding your specific situation.

Library of Congress Cataloging-in-Publication Data:

Loo, Marcus H.
    The prostate cancer sourcebook : how to make informed
treatment choices / Marcus H. Loo, and Marian Betancourt.
        p.   cm.
    Includes index.
    ISBN 0-471-15927-1 (pbk. : alk. paper)
    1. Prostate–Cancer–Popular works.   I. Betancourt, Marian.
    II. Title.
    RC280.P7L66   1998
    616.99'463–dc21   97-33001

Printed in the United States of America.

10 9 8 7 6 5 4 3 2 1

To Donna, Christopher, and Courtney.
M.L.

To Tom and Mary Ellen, Karen and Dan, Hilary and Julia.
M.B.

Contents

Introduction   xv

Part One
Discovery

1 A Primer on the Prostate   **3**
The Mechanics of the Prostate   5
The Geography of the Prostate   7
The Role of Hormones   7

2 Diseases of the Prostate   **9**
Benign Prostatic Hyperplasia (BPH)   10
Symptoms of BPH   13
Treatment for BPH   15
Prostatitis   20
Prostatic Intraepithelial Neoplasia (PIN)   21

3 How Prostate Cancer Develops   **23**
Symptoms of Prostate Cancer   24
Metastatic Cancer   25

4 Understanding the Risk Factors   **28**
Aging   29
Family History   29
Race   30
Environment and Diet   31
Unproved Risk Factors   35

Part Two
Guidelines for Diagnosis and Staging

5 Diagnostic Tests   **39**

Digital Rectal Examination (DRE)   39

Clinical Biopsy   41

Other Staging Tests   43

The Cost of Screening   45

Questions to Ask About Screening   46

6 The Controversial PSA Test   **48**

How PSA Is Measured   49

Adjusting for Age and Race   50

Adjusting for Density and Velocity   51

Screening Dilemmas   52

7 Grading and Staging   **54**

The Gleason Score   54

The TNM System   55

Staging   56

Health Insurance and Biopsy   58

Part Three
Treatment for Early Localized Prostate Cancer

8 Watchful Waiting   **63**

Controversy of Early Treatment   64

Degrees of Difference in Early Cancer   65

9 Surgery: Radical Prostatectomy   **68**

Technique of Radical Prostatectomy   69

Risks of Prostatectomy   73

Lymphadenectomy: Removing Lymph Nodes   75

Pathology of the Prostate Specimen   76

The Risk of Recurrence   79

Questions to Ask About Surgery   79

10 Before and After Surgery   82
The Weeks Before Surgery   82
Things to Do Before Surgery: A Checklist   89
The Day and Night Before Surgery   90
The Day of Surgery   91
After Surgery   93
Before You Go Home: A Checklist   97

11 External Beam Radiation Therapy   99
How It Works   101
Short-Term Side Effects   104
Long-Term Side Effects   105
Combination Therapies   106
Follow-Up Care   107
The Radiation Treatment Team   108
The Cost of Radiation Therapy   109

12 Brachytherapy (Interstitial Radiation)   111
The Procedure   112
Complications   115
Short-Term Side Effects of Implants   116
Questions to Ask About Radiation Therapy   117

Part Four
Treatment for Advanced Prostate Cancer

13 Hormonal Therapy for Metastatic Cancer   121
Why Cells Become Immune to Treatment   123
Orchiectomy   124
Synthetic Hormones   124
Maximal Androgen Blockade (MAB)   127
Other Strategies   128
Managing Hormone-Refractory Cancer   128
The Cost of Treatment   131

Part Five
Making the Decision

14 Choosing Physicians and a Treatment Center   **135**
Finding a Urologist   135
Comprehensive Cancer Treatment Centers   137
Support Services at Treatment Centers   138
Paying for Treatment   140

15 Nonmedical Aids to Treatment   **143**
Support from Family and Friends   144
In the Workplace   144
Support Groups   145
Private Counseling   146
Reducing the Stress of Living with Cancer   147

16 Making Your Decision   **150**
Getting More Medical Opinions   152
Considering Your Other Medical Conditions   154
Considering Your Emotional Response   154
Sharing Decision Making with Your Family   155
Proximity to Treatment Centers   156
The Cost of Treatment   157

Part Six
Recovery

17 Coping with Temporary Incontinence   **161**
Functioning with a Catheter   163
Strengthening the External Sphincter   164
Using Protective Products   166
Treating Severe Incontinence   166

18 Restoring Potency After Prostate Cancer   **168**
The Mechanics of an Erection   170
Treatment Options   170
Vacuum Erection Device (VED)   171

Transurethral Therapy 172
Pharmacologic Erection Program (PEP) 174
Penile Prostheses 176
The Cost of Treatment 177

19 Monitoring Your Health **178**
PSA Surveillance 178
Staying Healthy 182
The Future for You and Your Family 184

Appendix 1 Information Resources **187**

Appendix 2 Selected Studies **194**

Appendix 3 Bibliography **197**

**Appendix 4 Sources of Financial Aid for Screening
and Treatment** **199**

Appendix 5 What to Know About Medical Insurance **201**

Appendix 6 Your Right to Medical Records **207**

Appendix 7 Americans with Disabilities Act **208**

Appendix 8 Prostate Cancer Clinical Trials **211**

Appendix 9 Glossary **215**

Index **223**

Acknowledgments

Our sincere thanks to the physicians and health care professionals who shared their expertise on prostate cancer treatment and patient care including John Wei, M.D., James Wong, M.D., Peter Farano, M.D., J. François Eid, M.D., John W. Coleman, M.D., John H. McGovern, M.D., and E. Darracott Vaughn, M.D., chairman of the Department of Urology, the New York Hospital–Cornell University Medical Center. Special thanks and appreciation to literary agent Vicky Bijur.

Introduction

It has been said that prostate cancer is as much a philosophy as it is a disease. It is the only cancer offering such a variety of treatment options and the only cancer where doing nothing at all might sometimes be the wisest "treatment" choice. Some prostate cancer is so slow-growing that in some cases old age may kill first.

For African American men, prostate cancer is the leading cancer killer. For all other races, it is the second leading cancer killer after lung cancer. In 1996, more than 300,000 men were diagnosed with prostate cancer in the United States. More than 40,000 died of it. A boy born today in the United States has approximately a 13 percent chance of developing prostate cancer in his lifetime.

Although we cannot yet prevent prostate cancer, or cure it except with early detection, we have made enormous progress in the 1990s with more sophisticated surgical techniques, state-of-the-art radiation technology, and hormonal drugs. Some very exciting research is in progress and we are hopeful that we are getting closer to a better understanding of this enigmatic disease.

Perhaps the most exciting development in the 1990s has been the ability to identify prostate cancer with a simple blood test of one of the most specific tumor markers known. This remarkable test detects the level of prostate-specific antigen (PSA) present in the blood. This substance is produced by the prostate in every man and the level in the blood increases when something disrupts or irritates the prostate—either cancer or a benign condition. A high PSA level indicates the possible need for a prostate biopsy, which is how prostate cancer is often discovered. Before the discovery of this test, prostate cancer could not be detected until it was clinically apparent or discovered with a digital rectal examination. By then, the cancer was generally advanced, and the only treatment choice was hormonal therapy to slow the disease for as long as possible.

Ironically, this ability to find prostate cancer early enough to cure it has created enormous controversy about screening and treatment protocols. Because more prostate cancer is now diagnosed and treated based on biochemical information (the PSA test) rather than clinical symptoms, "overtreatment" is a major concern. The incidence of histologic or "latent" cancer exceeds clinical cancer by eight times. Nearly a third of American men will have this latent prostate cancer by the time they are 50—many years before the cancer becomes clinically evident or creates symptoms. This means they can choose to have their prostate and the cancer removed and risk possible impotence and urinary incontinence, or they can leave it there and wait and see what happens. What an agonizing predicament. How can a man decide what to do? Will the cancer grow slowly over his lifetime, or will it be a highly aggressive type that will grow fast and kill him?

The medical establishment has to ask itself if it is wise to tell men they have a cancer that may never cause them problems. They may be perfectly happy without this information. Autopsy studies have shown that almost all men over 90 have prostate cancer that was never recognized. Should all men over 50 have the PSA test and digital rectal examination? No consensus has been achieved concerning widespread screening for prostate cancer because it has not been proven that screening for prostate cancer alters overall survival. The only justification for universal screening is to save lives. These issues fuel the current controversy about the proper management of prostate cancer, as well as guidelines for screening for the disease.

Generally, prostate cancer is a relatively slow-growing disease with estimated doubling times of between 2 and 4 years, which is the time it takes for one cancer cell to become two, or for one million to become two million. In contrast, most other malignancies, such as breast, lung, and colon cancer, generally have faster doubling times, one of weeks or months (although researchers recently reported that certain types of breast cancer may have a slow doubling time, too). Ironically, while prostate cancer is slow to grow, it is also a very stubborn cancer that resists chemotherapy and eventually resists the beneficial effects of hormone therapy in men who have widespread metastatic disease.

With most other cancers, the goal of treatment is to kill or remove the disease. But with prostate cancer this is not always the case. Because it is slow-growing, a decision can be made on whether to treat or not to treat, as well as what kind of treatment to choose. The treatment options available to a 50-year-old man may be very different from those that would be best for an 80-year-old. In addition to the difference in life expectancy, each man's disease may have very different growth patterns and characteristics. The younger man may want to seek more aggressive therapy, because even if the prostate cancer is very slow-growing, it may reach the point at which it will someday escape the confines of the prostate and spread to other organs.

Prostate cancer is a disease of aging. The longer the prostate is exposed to androgens—the male hormones—the greater the risk of cancer. This situation is similar to many kinds of breast cancer, in which the breast ducts become sites for cellular changes caused by the long-term exposure to estrogen.

The recent discovery of a prostate cancer gene suggests a genetic connection, but this link pertains to only a small percentage of the men who get prostate cancer. Diet and the environment are also suspected of having an effect, because prostate cancer is much more common in Western industrialized populations with diets high in animal fat. Interestingly, the dog is the only animal that gets prostate cancer. Is this perhaps because the dog eats the same high-animal-fat, low-fiber diet?

There are racial differences, too. We know that more African American men die from prostate cancer than white men or Asians, but we are not sure if it is because more of them get the disease, or if it progresses faster in African Americans. The age-adjusted incidence of prostate cancer in African American men is about 50 percent higher than in white men. Interestingly, the lifetime cumulative probability of being diagnosed with prostate cancer is 10 percent for African Americans compared with 5 percent for white men. The cause of these differences is likely related to hereditary as well as environmental factors. Nutrition may contribute to the lower incidence of prostate cancer that exists in Asian compared to non-Asian populations.

Because many more men will die *with* prostate cancer than *from* it, a great deal of debate has centered on the diagnosis and treatment of prostate cancer in men without symptoms. The treatment options for early localized cancer include surgery to remove the prostate and the cancer, or radiation therapy to destroy the cancer cells, or doing nothing but monitoring to see what happens. There is hormonal treatment for advanced metastatic cancer. And there are treatment combinations.

The appeal of watchful waiting is obvious. You can stay where you are, spend no money, and continue to enjoy your sex life. Aggressive treatment is often unnecessary, especially given the risks of undesirable side effects. There are no hard-and-fast rules, but studies indicate that men in their 70s or 80s with a small, slow-growing, localized tumor are good candidates for this option. A man in his 70s needs to consider the stress of surgery or radiation and the risk of incontinence or impotence to remove a cancer that may never cause him any problems or shorten his life. If he has other conditions, such as heart disease, he needs to consider the combined effects on his lifestyle of his illnesses and the outcome of treatment. More aggressive treatment, such as radiation or surgery, can be started later, if the cancer begins to grow faster, although surgery could be ruled out if the cancer invades other organs. Before choosing to watchfully wait, the patient and his physician should be fairly confident that the prostate cancer cells are doubling at a slow rate and the volume of cancer is low.

Surgery to remove the prostate is the window of opportunity that once closed cannot be reopened. This is one of the most compelling reasons men make this treatment choice, because the "what ifs" are endless. What if the cancer spreads out of the prostate and surgery may no longer be an option? What if radiation scars the prostate and the cancer recurs? It may not be possible then to remove the prostate. Surgery also provides the opportunity to find out if the cancer has spread into the lymph nodes or other nearby organs.

Younger men with early localized cancer need to calculate the possible doubling time, or the odds for progression of the cancer. If they expect to live 30 more years, will the cancer grow fast enough to kill them? Most men in this situation choose to gamble on surgery and the possible aftereffects it may have on their potency and continence. We cannot say surgery is good for all men with prostate cancer, but it is definitely good for many.

We still have not proven that radical surgery has reduced the mortality rate from prostate cancer, although some studies will reach completion early in the 21st century. The number of surgeries done for early localized prostate cancer has mushroomed in the 1990s, and it will be many years before we know the survival rates for these men. Accurate rates of survival after surgery can only be determined in studies carried out for 10 to 15 years that compare men of similar cancer stage and grade, age, and race. Ignoring these factors has been a shortcoming of past clinical studies, when survival rates were based on studies of all men, regardless of these differences.

Radiation is often the choice of men with other conditions, such as heart or lung disease, that preclude surgery, and in men with more locally advanced disease. If the disease has already spread to the seminal vesicles or broken through the wall of the prostate, surgery is not a good option. Some younger men with localized cancer also prefer radiation over surgery. They gamble on the treatment knocking out most of the cancer and improving the odds that the cancer will not catch up to them before they die of old age.

Radiation treatment can be done in two ways: with an external beam delivered over a period of 6 to 8 weeks, or by implanting radioactive seeds into the prostate. This procedure is known as brachytherapy, and with recently improved capabilities of placing the seeds more accurately, this treatment has become more popular. For external beam therapy, proximity to a treatment center is a primary consideration because daily treatments for almost two months are necessary. Brachytherapy is currently done in only a few medical centers, so proximity to one of these centers is a factor in choosing a treatment plan.

The risk of impotence from injured nerves that can occur with surgery is not present with radiation, but there is a risk with external beam radiation of the blood vessels needed for erection becoming so scarified that they do not deliver enough blood to the penis. Radiation is also used as palliative treatment to reduce pain in more advanced cases of prostate cancer. It is sometimes used after surgery as adjuvant treatment if the cancer is found to have extended beyond the prostate or into the seminal vesicles.

Hormone therapy is not a cure for prostate cancer. It seeks to slow down the progression of metastatic disease in men who are not candidates for surgery or radiation therapy. Hormone therapy blocks the body's production of male hormones primarily from the testicles. This can be accomplished with the surgical removal of the testicles, which few men choose, or with drugs, now the most common form of hormonal treatment.

Although hormonal therapy has increased survival time for men with advanced stages of prostate cancer, we still do not know why some prostate cancer cells become resistant to this treatment, or how long it will take them to become resistant—that is, hormone refractory—because men respond differently. This subject is the focus of a great deal of study, and many clinical trials indicate we are learning more about hormonal treatment of prostate cancer. There is always hope of an imminent breakthrough.

Combinations of treatment are often prescribed for advanced prostate cancer. Hormonal therapy is sometimes used prior to surgery (neoadjuvant therapy) to shrink the tumor and downstage the disease in an attempt to make it easier to remove all of the cancer. There is currently much controversy as to whether this treatment really works with surgery. It is usually more successful with radiation, because when the radiation beam has a smaller target, it is less likely to affect other organs. Hormonal therapy is also used as an adjuvant therapy after surgery or radiation if the chance of local recurrence is high.

Chemotherapy is not used in the treatment of prostate cancer because it does not seem to work. With other cancers, chemotherapy can be an effective systemic treatment—that is, it treats the entire body—to wipe out cancer cells. Medications used for traditional chemotherapy are cytotoxic drugs—drugs that kill cells. For some reason, these drugs do not kill prostate cancer cells effectively. However, chemotherapy is sometimes used on prostate cancer patients when the disease has metastasized to other organs, and this treatment can either slow the spread of the disease or reduce the bothersome symptoms such as bone pain.

Cryosurgery is still investigational and few physicians use it. This treatment is rarely covered by health insurance. It uses subzero temperatures to destroy cancer cells, most commonly in men who have had radiation treatment without success. Although cryosurgery is less invasive than traditional surgery and requires a shorter hospital stay, the long-term effectiveness is unknown. Complications are high, including a 50- to 75-percent risk of impotence.

There is no single treatment for prostate cancer that is right for all men. Furthermore, it is not just the cancer itself that must be considered. Treatment decisions depend on physical health, emotional ability to deal with changes, support system and family, and available medical treatment facilities. Some men make their decisions based solely on the "scientific" evidence, that is, the size and stage of the cancer, while others take a more dimensional approach.

One elderly Chinese man told me he would not like to have surgery because he might become a burden to his family if there were complications from surgery and he were left incontinent. Like many Chinese families, several generations live, and often work, together. My patient believed that caring for him would mean a family member would be taken away from work. I identified strongly with his thinking, although I suspected that his family would not object to taking care of him if necessary. My elderly patient also reminded me that he considered surgery a "Western" concept, and that in China, surgery is rarely used as a treatment option for prostate cancer. This man chose radiation therapy not because he believed it to be the best treatment for his cancer—he believed it was the best treatment for *him!*

Impotence as a side effect of prostate cancer treatment is the biggest emotional hurdle for many men, which is clearly illustrated in the case of a 61-year-old patient of mine who discovered prostate cancer through his routine annual physical exam. His PSA test was above normal and a biopsy revealed that he had prostate cancer. Suddenly his world crashed. He was a university professor and truly loved his work. He was also crazy about his wife with whom he had a vigorous and romantic sex life. The thought of that changing because of prostate cancer treatment clearly had him in a panic. He was also very angry and at first refused to believe he had cancer.

During his weeks of agonizing about what to do, *Time* magazine published a cover story of General Norman Schwartzkopf, who had also recently discovered prostate cancer through a routine blood test. Subsequently, Andy Grove, chief executive officer of Intel, wrote a story in *Fortune* magazine about his experience with radiation therapy. The editor Michael Korda was in the process of writing his book *Man to Man* about his experience with prostate cancer.

Well-known men who discovered their prostate cancer early helped make public the controversies about screening and treatment. As Korda put it, choosing the best treatment for prostate cancer was clearly "the decision from hell." There were other well-known men who did not know early enough, and some died (rock star Frank Zappa and actors Bill Bixby and Telly Savalas). Savalas lived in years of agony because he did not go to a doctor when he knew something was wrong.

My patient identified with the men who had recently made their prostate cancer diagnosis public and found some comfort in the way they had confronted this epidemic of prostate cancer. He was determined to find a way to cope. But it was his wife who had the most influence in making a decision about treatment. She convinced him that he was more important to her than their sex life, and if necessary, they would adapt to new ways of enjoying sex. They decided together on the nerve-sparing surgery. The treatment was successful, and there were no signs that the cancer had spread outside his prostate. Following surgery, he maintained continence, and gradually, over a period of many months, he was able to get an erection naturally.

The side effects of surgery, radiation, and hormone treatment vary in every man, which is why it is so important for you to learn all you can and participate fully in the management of your treatment and follow-up care. This book is arranged so that you can learn what you need to know about your prostate and prostate cancer, as well as the questions you need to ask, and what you must consider before you go forward with treatment.

The "Discovery" section includes a primer on the prostate with information on both benign and malignant conditions, as well as risk factors for prostate cancer. "Guidelines for Diagnosis and Staging" is a step-by-step guide that explains diagnostic tests. Even if you have already been diagnosed with prostate cancer, this screening section, especially the chapter on the controversial PSA blood test, will help you understand the effects of particular treatment options.

The "Treatment" sections provide information on options for early localized cancer, including watchful waiting, surgery, and radiation—both external beam and internal seed implantation. There are also chapters on treating metastatic cancer, as well as treating hormone refractory cancer.

The final section of the book offers help through your recovery with some advice on coping with temporary urinary incontinence, restoring potency (there have been many advancements in this therapy recently), staying healthy, and monitoring PSA. Several appendixes will help you locate sources of information and support, clinical trials, health insurance considerations, and financial aid for treatment. The glossary may help you understand some of the new language you will encounter in your voyage through treatment and recovery.

Prostate cancer is a very big issue and cannot really be addressed until you understand as much as you can about your particular disease. It cannot be confronted until you get more than one opinion, and until you take a good hard look at your own situation and your own temperament. You need to think about the kind of emotional support available to you, treatment centers and physicians, and what your medical insurance allows. All of these factors play a role in your decision.

It is vitally important for you to be well informed about how your prostate functions, how prostate cancer develops in your body, what the various treatment options will accomplish, how treatment will affect the quality of your life, and how your physicians make decisions about your treatment. Keep in mind that physicians have biases, too. A radiation oncologist would naturally consider his or her treatment better, whereas a urologist might lean toward surgery. Although I am a urologist, I have tried to keep my own bias out of this book and I ask you to consider all the options available.

By walking you through the process of prostate cancer treatment and recovery, I hope you will be able to gain a perspective on the current treatment available as well as the controversies on this very unusual cancer. This book is meant to guide you through the diagnosis and treatment of prostate cancer and help you find out what you need to know to make the best decision for your particular disease, then move on with your life.

PART ONE

Discovery

1

A Primer on the Prostate

On an episode of the popular television drama, *ER,* a doctor chided his newly divorced colleague for failing to take advantage of the sexual opportunities of the single life. "The prostate doesn't last forever," he quipped.

Most men don't really know how long the prostate lasts, or what exactly it does, for that matter. Indeed they are often unaware of its existence until problems begin. Some mistakenly call it their *prostrate,* which may be an appropriate word to describe how they feel when they have chronic problems with their prostate. Most do know, however, that the prostate has to do with sex and if it is removed it could ruin their sex life as they know it. This is a compelling fear, and probably the reason why so many men never seek treatment for prostate problems, even those brought on by the ordinary and natural condition of aging.

The prostate is a gland of the male reproductive tract; its primary role is to produce seminal fluid. It sits like a doughnut at the base of the bladder with the urethra passing through the hole of the doughnut. The urethra carries urine or ejaculate out through the penis. The rectum lies directly behind the prostate, and it is this back part of the prostate that can be reached by the doctor during a digital rectal examination (DRE).

When a male child is born, his prostate gland is about the size of a pea and weighs 1 gram, which is a fraction of an ounce. There are two spurts of growth in the prostate. The first occurs at puberty, until it matures at around age 20 and is the size of a walnut. It weighs 15 to 20 grams. Another growth spurt occurs when a man is in his 40s or 50s. This enlargement is known as benign prostatic hyperplasia (BPH), which is explained in the next chapter. By the time a man is 70 or 80, his prostate can weigh 30 to 60 grams or more. Some men have prostates bigger than an apple.

3

The prostate is made of smooth muscle, and spongy glandular and fibrous tissue. The glands are lined with cells that secrete fluid, which is deposited in the urethra during ejaculation through a system of branching ducts. The smooth muscle and fibrous tissue are interwoven between the glandular tissue, much the way the glands and milk ducts are interwoven in the female breast. In middle age, or when the prostate begins to enlarge, it is the smooth muscle and connective tissue known as the *stroma* that increases in volume. The most striking feature of BPH enlargement is this stromal outgrowth.

Seminal vesicles, which look like two clusters of tiny grapes, lie on either side of the prostate. These glands produce the sticky secretion that gives semen its consistency and about 60 percent of its volume. The substance

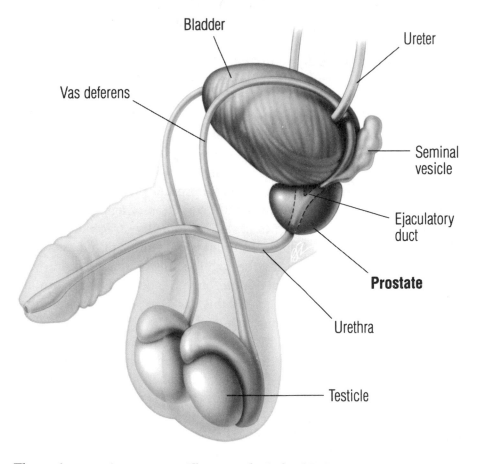

The male reproductive tract. *Illustration by Richard LaRocca.*

contains sugars, minerals, and enzymes to help sperm survive in the female reproductive tract.

The *vas deferens,* two thick, muscular tubes, about 18 inches long, connect each testicle to the prostate and function as ducts to get the sperm from the testicles to the ejaculatory duct of the prostate. These tubes are divided during a vasectomy, so that sperm can no longer pass into the semen. A vasectomy is a highly effective form of male contraception.

A network of nerves and blood vessels surround the prostate like a hair net, and these are sometimes injured or severed in the surgical removal of the prostate, causing impotence. There are two *neurovascular bundles* on either side of the prostate. These are sheaths containing the critical nerves that help mediate erection. Science still cannot explain exactly what causes an erection, but we know that the nerves tell the arteries to dilate and take more blood into the erectile bodies of the penis. When blood fills the penis and is trapped there, the penis becomes engorged, and thus erect. The vital nerves involved in this hydraulic system run along either side of the prostate.

These neurovascular bundles lie against the prostate and can also be the site of cancer cells escaping from the prostate. Because of their proximity to the gland itself, it is a very tricky surgical maneuver to keep these sheaths out of harm's way during surgery. The nerve-sparing surgical technique of radical prostatectomy seeks to do this. Radiation treatment can cause the nerves and blood vessels to become calloused or scarified and no longer able to carry blood into the penis. Thus, radiation therapy may also cause impotence.

The Mechanics of the Prostate

This small but complex gland has many tasks to carry out in its primary function to support and promote male insemination and fertility. It is a factory for production of nutrient-rich seminal fluid to help transport sperm from the testicles out of the body during ejaculation and to help the sperm survive in the female reproductive tract. It is a gatekeeper, or valve, that allows sperm and urine to flow in the right direction through the urethra. A ring of muscles near the neck of the bladder—the internal sphincter—clamps down during ejaculation to prevent semen from backing up into the bladder. If this mechanism is damaged, retrograde ejaculation or backup of semen into the bladder may result. The prostate is also a pump during orgasm, contracting the muscles to force semen into the urethra. Retrograde ejaculation occurs in 50 percent of men who undergo a transurethral resection of the prostate (TURP) for BPH because the bladder neck and internal sphincter are typically resected during the procedure. There is more on this subject in Chapter 2.

Sperm and Seminal Fluid

Sperm from the testicles is transported by the vas deferens to the ejaculatory duct, which runs through the prostate. Sperm is then mixed with fluid from the prostate and seminal vesicles to form the ejaculate. More than half of the ejaculate comes from the seminal vesicles and 15 to 30 percent from the prostate gland. Sperm from the testicles makes up about 5 percent of the ejaculate volume.

When semen is ejaculated into the vagina, it exists as a semisolid gel that forms a plug on the female cervix. The plug serves as an efficient delivery system for sperm trapped in the seminal coagulant. The gel spontaneously liquefies after 10 to 15 minutes due to the presence of an enzyme known as prostate-specific antigen (PSA), a protein that is produced by the prostate gland. This protein molecule can also enter the bloodstream in greater amounts when something is wrong. Any process that disrupts the normal ductal structure of the prostate, such as prostate cancer, BPH, or prostatitis (inflammation), will cause more PSA to leak into the blood. Therefore, when serum PSA is elevated, it suggests a process in the prostate is disrupting its normal ductal architecture. (See Chapter 6 for more information about PSA.)

The seminal fluid also contains minerals (e.g., zinc) and sugar (e.g., fructose), as well as other enzymes and nutrients, that sperm need to survive in the female reproductive tract. It is believed that prostate fluid also serves in some antibacterial capacity and that elderly men with chronic bacterial inflammation of the prostate (prostatitis) have reduced antibacterial activity as well as reduced prostatic zinc levels. Nevertheless, studies with zinc supplements have failed to confirm the efficacy of dietary zinc as protection against the recurrence of prostatitis.

When the prostate is removed, no seminal fluid is produced—that is, there is no emission during sexual climax. However, this change does not affect the ability for sexual arousal and orgasm. Erection, orgasm, and ejaculation are three separate events, but usually are coordinated to occur together. Ejaculation and orgasm may still occur with impotence or erectile dysfunction.

Despite its complex role, the prostate is not a vital organ like the heart or lungs. Men can live without it, although given a choice, most would rather not.

The Geography of the Prostate

For diagnostic purposes, the prostate is divided into three major zones. Knowing the geography of the prostate can help in understanding how symptoms develop when something is wrong.

The *peripheral zone,* or the outside of the prostate, accounts for about 70 percent of the glandular tissue of the prostate, which is the site of most prostate cancer. This area is directly behind the rectum, part of which the doctor can touch during a DRE.

The *transition zone* is the small inner core that surrounds the urethra. This zone accounts for about 5 percent of the prostate's volume early on, but with age, this area gets larger. This noncancerous enlargement of the prostate (BPH) begins after age 40 in all men. The enlarged tissue may cause a pinching off of the urethra or obstruction, leading to urination problems with advancing age. Although the transition zone is where urinary problems often begin, it accounts for only a small percent of prostate cancer.

The *central zone* comprises about 25 percent of the prostate's volume and is sandwiched between the peripheral and transitional zones. It is the least likely site for prostate cancer.

There is also muscle and fibrous tissue in the front section of the prostate where no glandular tissue is present–the fibromuscular zone. The term *lobe* is also used to describe the right and left sections of the prostate gland, and a tumor may develop in one or both lobes.

The Role of Hormones

Testosterone is an essential player in prostate cancer. This hormone–or androgen, as male hormones are labeled–is produced mainly by the testicles. It can produce prostate cancer in rats that are given large doses. However, while all men produce testosterone, not all men get prostate cancer. Interestingly, men who have testicles damaged or removed prior to puberty never get prostate cancer or BPH.

The prostate grows rapidly during puberty because it is fed by androgens, which make it possible for the prostate to produce seminal fluid. Androgens also stimulate the development of body hair, deepen the voice, and increase muscle bulk in the upper body. The primary androgen is testosterone, but some androgens are produced by the adrenal glands that lie above each kidney. Briefly, here is how the process works:

1. The hypothalamus, a small gland at the base of the brain, produces luteinizing hormone-releasing hormone (LHRH).

2. LHRH acts on the nearby pituitary gland to produce luteinizing hormone (LH) and follicle-stimulating hormone (FSH).

3. FSH acts on certain cells of the testicles to produce sperm.

4. LH acts on the Leydig cells of the testicles to produce testosterone, the primary male androgen.

5. An enzyme, 5-alpha reductase, converts testosterone to its active metabolite and more potent form, dihydrotestosterone (DHT).

6. DHT diffuses into prostate cells to influence growth such as the development of benign prostatic hyperplasia (BPH).

7. Adrenocorticotropic hormone (ACTH) is produced by the pituitary gland to act on the adrenal glands to produce other androgens that may also influence prostate growth.

While these androgens nourish the prostate, they can also nourish prostate cancer cells. Testosterone, for example, is responsible for cell division in the prostate, just as estrogen may be responsible for the growth of breast cancer. The enlargement of the prostate in middle age may be caused by the complex relationship of aging and hormones, although this connection does not always lead to prostate cancer.

2

Diseases of the Prostate

The prostate of every man begins to enlarge in middle age and this enlargement is the primary cause of the need to urinate more often. The first wave of 76 million baby boomers in the United States turned 50 in 1996. The total male population over 50 will nearly double by the year 2020, and primary care physicians and urologists will see more men with symptoms from enlarged prostates. At age 50, a prostate weighs from 30 to 100 grams (1 to $3^1/2$ ounces) and is much larger than it was at age 20. There are approximately 15 million men in the United States with symptoms of benign prostatic hyperplasia (BPH) and the vast majority are not seeking treatment.

More than half the men over 60 have some degree of BPH, and by the time they are 80, most men have the disease. BPH is one of two noncancerous conditions of the prostate whose symptoms are sometimes confused with prostate cancer. The other is prostatitis, an inflammatory condition.

It is ironic that although the prostate is primarily concerned with sexual reproduction, when something goes wrong, it more frequently causes problems with urination. Because the prostate surrounds the urethra, an 8-inch-long tube extending from the neck of the bladder through the prostate and penis, any change in the prostate's size can affect the dynamics of urinary flow. This close proximity to the urethra and bladder make it a crucial link in the efficient flow of urine. For example, as the prostate enlarges, the space around the urethra–the hole of the doughnut–gets pinched off or blocked. The enlarged prostate gland squeezes on the urethra the way a fist would squeeze on a straw. In extreme cases it can close off the passage altogether and impede the flow of urine.

Benign Prostatic Hyperplasia (BPH)

In BPH the inner core of prostate tissue—the transition zone that surrounds the urethra—expands from the proliferation of cells. This cell division is called *hyperplasia*. The enlargement of the prostate tissue and the reduction in the size of the doughnut hole cause problems with urination or ejaculation because of the pressure on the urethra. These same symptoms can be signs of cancer, but with cancer the symptoms usually develop more insidiously. The benign condition of BPH does not increase the risk of cancer. However, both conditions can exist simultaneously, so screening for prostate cancer and treatment for symptomatic BPH is always important. Therefore, the natural processes of the prostate must be understood.

Because BPH develops on the inside core, or the transition zone, of the prostate, it cannot generally be detected with a digital rectal exam (DRE). Only about half the men with microscopic BPH develop prostate enlargement that can be felt with a DRE. The 50 percent of men who develop enlargement to this degree may need surgery to remove the excess tissue from the inner core to relieve the pressure on the urethra. According to some studies, approximately 25 percent of all men will require treatment for their symptoms of BPH if they live to be 80. A 60-year-old man has a 60 percent chance of developing microscopic BPH and a 25 percent cumulative chance of requiring surgery. With the advent of new pharmacological ways to treat BPH, this cumulative risk of needing surgery has significantly decreased.

The natural history of BPH is highly variable and currently we don't have good data over time about how patients do with or without treatment. And we don't know if diet or race are contributing factors. Size or volume of the BPH tissue is different insofar as Asians have smaller prostates in general, but they develop symptoms with similar frequency, so size is not the important feature by itself.

It does appear in some men that the symptoms may not progress. Between 50 and 60 percent of patients studied with BPH either stabilized or had spontaneous improvement over time. This lack of data explains the lack of uniformity of surgical treatment in the United States. There are few absolute indications for intervention and many men with symptoms do not require surgical treatment to remove the excessive tissue growth.

Although the cause of BPH is not completely understood, it is clearly related to aging and the presence of functioning testicles. A number of clinical and experimental observations attest to this fact. It has been known since the 1800s that removal of the testes results in shrinkage of prostate tissue and clinical improvement of symptoms of BPH. If a boy's testicles are removed prior to puberty, the boy never develops BPH or prostate cancer later in life.

In the early 1970s, Dr. Julianne Imperato-McGinley of Cornell University Medical College noticed an interesting genetic syndrome in a population of male infants from the Dominican Republic known as congenital 5-alpha reductase deficiency. This enzyme converts testosterone to the more potent androgen, dihydrotestosterone (DHT). Boys with this recessive genetic disorder lack the enzyme, and so the prostate does not grow normally. At birth, these children have a small phallus, and in adulthood the prostate remains small. Some tissues of the body respond to testosterone itself whereas others such as the prostate require DHT for growth and differentiation. These males are otherwise normal and have no sexual problems. From this observation it is clear that DHT and not testosterone is necessary for BPH development. BPH cannot develop without DHT. Medications that block the conversion of testosterone to DHT are often used to treat men with symptoms of BPH.

Ultimate regulation of the development of BPH occurs in the brain's control center in the interaction of the hypothalamus and pituitary glands. The hypothalamus releases a hormone known as luteinizing hormone releasing hormone (LHRH) that stimulates the pituitary gland to release luteinizing hormone (LH). LH travels in the blood and reaches the testicles where testosterone is produced. Testosterone is converted in the prostate epithelial cells to DHT by the enzyme 5-alpha reductase. DHT in turn combines with receptors in the nucleus of the prostate epithelial cells to produce cell growth and proliferation.

The paradox is that hormones diminish slightly as men age, yet the hormones are responsible for the increased cell proliferation that causes BPH. Normal growth and function of the prostate is dependent on androgens maintaining a balance between cell growth and cell death.

PSA and BPH

The presence of BPH does not mean prostate cancer is present or will develop. However, BPH may cause the prostate-specific antigen (PSA) level to rise. This rise may be from the BPH alone, or it may be an early indication of cancer, so it must be seriously explored. The frequent existence of clinically hidden or latent prostate cancer in men with BPH is well known. It is standard procedure when doing surgical treatment for BPH for a pathologist to microscopically examine any tissue that is removed. From 10 to 20 percent of men who undergo prostatectomy for BPH through a transurethral resection of the prostate (TURP) will be found to have microscopic prostate cancer usually of small volume and low grade. Thus, with more and more men electing to have nonsurgical treatment for BPH, physical exams and blood tests are imperative, so that occult cancer can be diagnosed before it causes symptoms or becomes more advanced.

Treatment with certain medications for BPH can also affect PSA. Proscar (finasteride) is a 5-alpha reductase inhibitor and decreases the DHT levels in men with BPH. When used to treat men with symptomatic BPH, Proscar will decrease the rate of growth of BPH tissue and generally cause a reduction in prostate volume. However, Proscar is known to decrease the PSA value in half after 6 months of therapy. For example, if a man's PSA level is 3.0 nanograms per milliliter (ng/ml) before beginning treatment with Proscar, and after 6 months of treatment the level decreases to 1.6, he should double that figure to 3.2 to learn his exact PSA level.

The Dynamic and Static Prostate

The urethral obstruction caused by BPH comes from both a dynamic and a static mechanical component. The dynamic obstruction is due to the tone of the smooth muscle (stroma) and its ability to relax and contract, whereas the static or mechanical element is simply the presence of the large bulky prostate pressing on the urethra and causing outlet obstruction.

The dynamic and static components vary widely in men. Some men with a small prostate may have a dynamic obstruction—that is, the muscles of the bladder neck and prostate do not relax adequately. On the other hand, in men with larger prostates, the static component may be more predominant in causing symptoms of BPH based on a more significant mass effect causing outlet obstruction.

The symptoms of BPH are highly variable and most men are relatively symptom-free. Symptoms are caused by obstruction of the urethra and alterations in bladder function. The size of the prostate is not always a predictor of the type or severity of symptoms. Some men with very large prostates have minimal symptoms, whereas others with relatively small glands are very symptomatic. Reasons for this paradox are incompletely understood but are believed to be due to relative contributions of the dynamic and static components.

During voiding, urine flows from the bladder through the urethra. In a prostate with BPH, the urethra is narrowed by mechanical obstruction of the enlarged prostate or by the dynamic obstruction of increased smooth muscle tone. The bladder tries to compensate for this increased resistance by generating a stronger bladder contraction to force out the urine. Over time, the bladder muscle is unable to compensate for the increasing outlet resistance and it fatigues, giving rise to the inability to completely empty the bladder and the possibility of leakage and incontinence. Imagine a stretched elastic band. If it is stretched a little and released, it returns to its original shape. However, if it is stretched to a considerably longer length, kept stretched, and then released, it eventually loses its elasticity and fails to return to its original shape. Similarly, the bladder can lose its capacity to empty itself of urine if it is chronically obstructed and overstretched. The retention of urine in the bladder can lead to urinary tract infection as well as formation of bladder stones, and in more severe cases, kidney failure can result from longstanding obstruction.

Symptoms of BPH

The symptoms of BPH are broadly classified as obstructive or irritative. Irritative symptoms include an increased need and urgency to urinate, especially the need to get up during the night (nocturia), and a burning sensation (dysuria) upon urinating. In extreme cases, BPH can cause incontinence.

Obstructive symptoms are a result of the bladder muscle's inability to overcome the outlet obstruction. Symptoms include a poor and slow stream of urine, a feeling of incompletely emptying the bladder, dribbling at the end of urination, an interruption of flow, and hesitancy or an inability to initiate urinary flow easily. Men with BPH may also develop blood in the urine due to bursting of dilated blood vessels at the bladder neck or surface of BPH tissue. Some have obstructive and irritative voiding symptoms whereas others "silently" develop chronic renal dysfunction and urinary tract infections. Some men have no real symptoms or complaints until these complications develop.

Whether irritative or obstructive, symptoms of BPH are subjective, highly variable, and unpredictable. The perplexing issue is the lack of relationship between prostate size and type and severity of voiding symptoms.

Because so many men do not seek medical help for the problem, they suffer in silence and may cope with their symptom by:

- Staying close to a bathroom at all times
- Reserving seats on the aisle wherever they go
- Wearing dark clothing to conceal leakage
- Taking frequent naps to make up for loss of sleep at night
- Curtailing social activities

Keep in mind that many of these symptoms are not unique to BPH and can also be caused by urinary tract infection, cancer, and neurological dysfunction. Such conditions must be carefully considered when there are BPH-like symptoms. Indications for treatment of BPH are not absolute, and given the vast array of medical and nonsurgical alternatives, it is important to have a very thorough workup with a urologist before deciding on treatment.

BPH Diagnosis

A complete BPH evaluation requires a very detailed history and physical examination, because the obstructive symptoms of BPH may also be due to other medical conditions such as stricture or scar tissue in the urethra, neurological conditions such as stroke, Parkinson's disease, or muscular sclerosis, which may affect bladder function by misinterpreting the brain's signals. Men who have had pelvic or abdominal surgery may often have injury to nerves that control bladder function. Urinary tract infection as well as stone disease and tumors of the bladder can bring on irritative symptoms and may often be confused with BPH.

A digital rectal exam (DRE) should be performed to assess the prostate as well as a urinalysis and urine culture to exclude the possibility of a urinary tract infection. Blood studies such as the serum PSA level and assessment of kidney function should be done. (See Chapter 5 for more information about diagnostic testing.)

If blood is found in the urine, either microscopically or if it is clearly visible, further evaluation is warranted. This should include an imaging study of the upper urinary tract with an intravenous pyelogram (IVP). A dye is given intravenously that is taken up by the kidneys and later excreted. When X-ray images are taken, the dye outlines the kidneys, ureters, and bladder. If an abnormality exists in the urinary tract, such as a stone or blockage to the kidneys, it can be clearly seen. An ultrasound of the kidney can also be used to determine the problem. (In some people the dye could cause an allergic reaction and the test should not be done.)

Evaluation of the lower urinary tract–the urethra and bladder–is done with a fiberoptic scope known as a cystoscope. Possible causes for blood in the urine (hematuria) other than BPH include the presence of stones in the kidney or bladder, prostate cancer, tumors of the kidney, ureter, or bladder, and congenital abnormalities of the urinary tract.

Part of the workup for BPH may often include a urinary flow rate determination. In this very simple test a patient with a full bladder is asked to urinate into a funnel connected to a measuring device that records the urine flow rate in milliliters per second. Then, with ultrasound it can be determined if any urine is left in the bladder after voiding. Men with severe BPH will often have a slow urinary flow rate and a moderate to high level of residual urine in the bladder.

Treatment for BPH

Before the development of new drug therapies, surgery was the primary treatment for BPH. With mild symptoms, watchful waiting is also an option for this benign condition. It was recognized years ago that approximately 50 to 60 percent of patients with BPH reach a certain level of symptoms and then stabilize or improve without any treatment. Only

1 to 2 percent of men who have BPH develop acute symptoms such as the inability to urinate.

Medications

BPH treatment protocols are in transition, with a decreased reliance on surgery and an increased interest in medical or pharmacological management. Many drugs may be used to affect growth of BPH tissue. These drugs may act on the pituitary (for example, to block LHRH), or to block the androgen receptor, or block the conversion of testosterone to DHT in the prostate. Finasteride (Proscar) is a 5-alpha reductase inhibitor. When taken orally, it prevents the conversion of testosterone to DHT.

Therapy with Proscar is directed at reducing the size or volume of the gland to improve urinary flow and symptoms and disrupting the progression of BPH by affecting the static or mechanical component of outlet obstruction. In clinical trials, men treated with finasteride for up to 12 months saw an approximately 20 percent reduction in prostate volume compared with men who did not take the medication.

Because it blocks some of the hormonal action that affects the prostate, this drug is also being studied for use as a possible prevention of prostate cancer in a large prostate cancer chemoprevention trial sponsored by the National Cancer Institute. (There is information about clinical trials in Appendix 8.)

There appear to be two locations for 5-alpha reductase activity: one in the prostate and the other in the middle layer of skin where the hair follicles are located. The Food and Drug Administration recently approved the use of finasteride to stimulate hair growth in balding.

Side Effects

Most men have few side effects with Proscar therapy and it does not generally interfere with their libido. However, in about 3 percent of patients on Proscar for more than 6 months, impotence, decreased libido, and a decrease in the volume of ejaculate may occur.

After 6 months of therapy with Proscar, the prostate not only shrinks but the medication reduces the PSA level by half. It is vital to understand this situation, because if a man is using the PSA test for annual screening for prostate cancer, the reading will be misleading. Thus, while using Proscar, it is necessary to double the PSA reading for a true value.

Other Pharmacological Treatment

Pharmacologic treatment with Proscar affects the static component of obstruction, and other medications such as alpha receptor blockers, for example, Hytrin (terazosin) and Cardura (doxazosin), treat the dynamic component of obstruction.

In men without BPH, the ratio of stromal to glandular tissue is 2 to 1. In men with BPH, the ratio is 5 to 1. Thus, BPH is primarily a stromal disease, and studies have found that the stromal tissue of the prostate gland and bladder neck area are richly endowed with alpha$_1$ adrenergic receptors that mediate the ability of the smooth muscle surrounding the prostate to contract and relax. These receptors are sparse in the body of the bladder, so it has been observed that drugs that would block the receptor would relax the smooth muscle and reduce the resistance in the bladder neck, thereby improving the flow of urine. The contractility of the bladder would not be affected because of the lack of alpha receptor innervation. This finding has led to the development of a number of alpha$_1$ adrenergic receptor blockers that may be used to medically manage patients with BPH.

Like all alpha$_1$ receptor blockers, these drugs can lower blood pressure and therefore are useful in treating hypertension as well. They are taken once a day, and unlike Proscar, have no significant effect on PSA. Side effects noted with these medications include dizziness, lightheadedness, fatigue, and sometimes impotence.

Surgical Treatment

With the inevitable development of BPH with advancing age, some men have severe enough bladder obstruction to warrant surgical treatment to open up the doughnut hole by cutting away some of the prostate tissue. The indications for this surgery include the inability to urinate, (acute urinary retention), renal failure, chronic obstruction, blood in the urine (hematuria), bladder stones, and recurrent urinary tract infections.

TURP is the second most common surgical procedure performed on men after cataract surgery. It accounts for about 40 percent of major surgical procedures performed by urologists at a cost to the health care system of $4 billion a year. With the focus of health care on cost containment, there is a great deal of incentive to develop nonsurgical alternatives for treating BPH, which has been achieved somewhat by the increased use of pharmacologic alternatives.

TURP removes some of the prostate tissue. Most commonly, tissue is removed from the transition zone surrounding the doughnut hole to widen the passageway and allow free flow of urine through the urethra. For obvious reasons, TURP is commonly known as the "Roto-Rooter" procedure. The entire gland is not removed during TURP, only the transition zone where BPH tissue develops. The peripheral zone is retained. However, if the prostate is very large, open abdominal surgery may be required to remove the bulky tissue. These surgical procedures are considered a form of prostatectomy, but they differ from a radical prostatectomy, which is the surgical removal of the entire prostate, a common treatment for localized prostate cancer.

TURP involves inserting a fiberoptic telescope through the urethra of the penis. The urologist can see and operate through this tube. Connected to this tube is the resectoscope, an electric device, which removes prostate tissue and cauterizes—seals—the blood vessels. Essentially, the instrument is used to make the hole of the doughnut larger and relieve pressure on the urethra. This procedure relieves urinary symptoms such as a weak stream or a sensation of incomplete bladder emptying. Treatment requires hospitalization from 1 to 3 days.

Although it is not used in the treatment of prostate cancer, TURP may sometimes relieve the symptoms caused by the cancer, such as pressure on the urethra. It may also be used as a biopsy method to check the tissue at the inner core or peripheral zone of the prostate. Tissue removed during the TURP procedure is routinely sent to a pathologist to check for the presence of prostate cancer. About 80 percent of cancers found this way are cured because the procedure removes all the cancerous tissue.

Prostate cancers found on pathological examination of TURP-removed tissue are known as transition zone cancers because the BPH tissue comes from that zone. These are generally of low grade and volume. There is a need for follow-up because the peripheral zone is still vulnerable, and this zone is not removed by TURP. Therefore, an annual DRE and PSA to monitor for prostate cancer are necessary.

Although not always successful, TURP was the most common surgical treatment for BPH before the development of medical therapies. It was recognized that 21 percent of patients treated with TURP were unsatisfied or did not improve, and 20 percent needed reoperation after 8 years due to regrowth of BPH tissue. Clearly, there was a need to identify beneficial alternatives to TURP.

The chance that symptoms will improve after TURP is from 75 to 95 percent compared with 60 to 85 percent with the alpha$_1$ receptor blockers, 50 to 70 percent with Proscar, and 30 to 50 percent with watchful waiting. Clearly TURP is the gold standard against which all nonsurgical alternatives must be compared.

Side Effects of TURP

From 5 to 10 percent of men may be impotent after TURP, 5 percent may experience urinary tract infections, and a few may be incontinent if the sphincter is damaged. (See Chapter 17 for information about coping with incontinence.)

Treatment with Microwaves

Alternatives to TURP have evolved in the 1990s. They include transurethral incision of the prostate, where an incision is made in the prostate but no tissue is removed. This procedure was popularized in Europe and is quite effective for patients with relatively small prostates. Laser therapy of the prostate or visual laser ablation of the prostate (VLAP) can also be done and carries less potential for complications than a TURP. More recently, the FDA approved the use of Prostatron microwave therapy for BPH. This procedure is done in the urologist's office and results so far have been encouraging.

Prostatron is a device that heats the enlarged prostate with microwaves. A catheter is threaded through the urethra into the prostate. A computer sends microwaves through the catheter to heat the prostate. This heat kills BPH tissue, which sloughs off, and pressure on the blocked urethra is relieved, accomplishing the same result as TURP. Cooling water circulates inside the catheter so that the patient does not feel the heat or get burned. Treatment with the Prostatron takes an hour, requires no anesthetic, and costs half as much as surgery. It has been used in 25 countries since 1991, and was approved by the Food and Drug Administration for use in the United States in 1996.

Prostatitis

Prostatitis is an inflammatory condition of the prostate that may or may not be caused by an infection. Infections of the prostate gland rarely occur before puberty, but they are common in adult men. Because many aspects of prostatitis are poorly understood, patients and doctors are often frustrated. Men will often have irritating or obstructive symptoms and their PSA will often be markedly elevated.

There are many different types of prostatitis. Acute bacterial prostatitis causes fever or chills as well as severe irritative and obstructive voiding symptoms, a general feeling of malaise, muscle aches and pains. When examined with a DRE, the prostate will feel very warm and soft. Urine analysis will show bacteria.

In chronic bacterial prostatitis, clinical features are more variable. The syndrome is unique, however, because of the persistence of bacteria in the prostate, which have not been fully treated and do not clear. Chronic bacterial prostatitis may feature recurrent urinary tract infections despite prior treatment with oral antibiotics.

Nonbacterial prostatitis is more common, but the cause is unknown.

Symptoms of Prostatitis

Prostatitis symptoms include painful urination, possibly a burning sensation, and the need to urinate frequently. There may be fever, blood in the urine, and less commonly lower back pain. Prostatitis also causes the PSA level to elevate—sometimes into the thousands. Irritation and obstruction are typically seen in men with BPH.

Treatment

Treatments may include antibiotics and medications to relax compression of the urethra. The choice of antibiotic must be tailored to the type of bacteria cultured from the urine. Typically, antibiotics are prescribed for up to 4 weeks or more.

Because most antibiotics taken orally achieve poor levels of concentration within the prostate, the bacteria in chronic prostatitis often persist after treatment. Symptoms may persist while repeat urine cultures fail to show any bacteria. Once the antibiotic is stopped, the bacteria regrow within the prostate and symptoms may worsen. Consequently, it is important to be on antibiotic therapy for a protracted period of time.

Prostatic Intraepithelial Neoplasia (PIN)

The search for clues to indicate the best approach for treating prostate cancer has focused on the microscopic changes referred to as high-grade prostatic intraepithelial neoplasia, or PIN. This microscopic finding is considered the most likely precursor of invasive cancer and is characterized by cellular proliferation within the prostate ducts and glands, known as atypia or dysplasia. PIN coexists with prostate cancer in more than 85 percent of cases. Therefore, the clinical importance of recognizing PIN is based on its strong association with invasive cancer. The identification of PIN alone in a prostate biopsy always warrants further search for invasive cancer.

PIN may develop decades before a cancer is detected. It is most often discovered when the PSA is higher than normal, indicating the need for biopsy and further screening. PIN is detected under the microscope in tissue removed with the needle biopsy. If it is low grade, there is no cause for alarm, but high-grade PIN calls for active surveillance, with periodic PSA tests and biopsies to watch for changes. Studies are in progress to determine if drugs can reverse the condition. Like other conditions of the prostate, PIN is most often related to aging. Whether PIN remains stable, regresses, or progresses is not yet clearly understood, but there is strong evidence that it can progress to invasive prostate cancer.

PIN has a very distinctive appearance and can only be diagnosed on biopsy. It is divided into three grades, with grade 1 being low and grades 2 and 3 being high. Patients with high-grade PIN should have biopsies periodically to look for cancer so that it can be detected early enough for curative treatment.

In some studies, up to 36 percent of patients who were identified with high-grade PIN in an initial biopsy were found to have prostate cancer on later biopsies. Autopsy studies show that the prevalence of

PIN and prostate cancer increase with age. Interestingly, there is a marked decrease in the prevalence and extent of high-grade PIN in men after hormonal therapy when compared with untreated patients. These findings suggest that prostate cells are hormone dependent. The decrease in PIN when androgens are blocked is believed to be caused by the acceleration of programmed cell death (apoptosis) and suggests that drugs such as Proscar may potentially be used to prevent the development of prostate cancer.

3

How Prostate Cancer Develops

There are two forms of prostate cancer: latent and clinical. Latent cancer shows no symptoms and is not detectable on physical exam, but a rising PSA level indicates the potential for the presence of cancer. (See Chapter 6 for a full explanation of PSA as a screening tool for prostate cancer.) Clinical cancer can be detected through a physical exam and has given rise to symptoms or complaints. It already exists in the form of a known carcinoma, a solid or self-contained tumor that can be seen or felt.

Cancer is really many different diseases. There are several major types of cancer and hundreds of subtypes. Lung cancer is very different from lymphoma or skin cancer. However, all cancers have in common the abnormal growth and division of cells. Deoxyribonucleic acid (DNA) is in the nucleus of each cell and this is where the genes are located.

The activity of human cells is controlled—or programmed—by DNA much the way software controls what a computer does. If the DNA programming runs amok for some reason, the genes lose control. It is as if the computer operator were hitting the command key over and over again without hitting the program key to give it direction. Cancer cells are normal cells that have developed the ability to multiply at an abnormal rate and are out of control. They do not attach to normal cells, but they do form abnormal groups and patterns. Cancer cells proliferate on their own and become autonomous. This is how they become *differentiated,* meaning they are forming abnormal groups and patterns of their own.

A cancer forming in a gland is called an adenocarcinoma, which accounts for 95 percent of prostate cancer. Most prostate cells are glandular cells that produce secretions. The prostate is made up of a system of ducts surrounded by fibrous tissue. A smaller portion of the prostate's cells make up the muscle and pumping activity. If the carcinoma is detected early enough, before it has spread out of the prostate capsule, it can potentially be cured.

Cancer is either in situ or invasive. *In situ* means "in place," contained within the gland. The cancer has not broken through the prostate wall into the surrounding soft tissue and fat. Invasive, or infiltrating, cancer can or already has broken through the ductal wall of the gland, perhaps penetrating the prostate capsule, seminal vesicles, blood vessels, and bladder, spreading (or metastasizing) to the lymph system or bones.

If the cancer is invasive, lymph nodes around the prostate will be examined during surgery, if performed, to find out if the cancer has begun to spread elsewhere. Lymphatic fluid flows through the body and the bean-shaped lymph nodes act like filters, catching what comes through the pipes. As part of the immune system, they filter out and get rid of foreign or abnormal cells. It is here that cancer cells are likely to travel first when they migrate from the prostate.

Prostate cancer is generally slow-growing and its *doubling time*—the time it takes to double in size from one cell to two, or one million to two million—could be years long, rather than weeks or months, as in some other cancers. About half of all prostate cancer takes more than 4 years to double in size, whereas some breast cancer doubles every 3 months, although recent studies have indicated there may also be some slow-growing breast cancers. Prostate cancer grows so slowly that in autopsy studies 80 percent of men who died of other causes after age 90 had latent prostate cancer unrecognized during their lifetime. Most prostate cancer typically develops as a lesion in the peripheral zone, so it is unlikely to cause urethral obstruction until it is advanced. The transition zone, which becomes obstructed when enlarged, is the site of only about 10 to 15 percent of prostate cancers.

Symptoms of Prostate Cancer

Early prostate cancer gives no warning at all. It is a characteristic of the disease that symptoms typically do not appear until the cancer is advanced. This is made clear by the fact that histologic cancer exceeds the presence of clinical cancer by as much as eight times. Prostate cancer cells grow for a long time before they become a tumor big enough to be detected by a DRE. But once they reach a certain critical mass or volume, prostate tumors can progress quickly. At this time, symptoms usually begin to appear and cancer cells may have already spread outside the prostate.

Commonly, local tumor growth in the prostate, whether it is benign or malignant, makes itself known by causing problems with urination, such as the need to urinate more often, having a sense of urgency, or having a weak stream. If the cancer has metastasized, the symptoms appear primarily in the bones. Prostate cancer can also be detected during a DRE by the change in the consistency, configuration, and symmetry of the prostate gland. Approximately 10 percent of men with voiding symptoms and no other clinical signs or symptoms of cancer have an occult (hidden) malignancy.

Obstructive and irritative symptoms are the most common symptoms of local cancer growth. When the cancer is the cause rather than the incidental finding of the local symptoms, it usually has appreciable mass and volume and is frequently not confined to the prostate.

Blood in the urine, or hematuria, is rarely associated with prostate cancer, but if it does occur, especially in an elderly man, this would suggest the need for further tests to look for cancer. Hematuria is an uncommon nonspecific sign in less than 15 percent of men with prostate cancer. Reasons for having blood in the urine involve local invasion of prostate cancer in the urethra or the base of the bladder. Renal failure may be a late manifestation of local spread once the cancer has invaded the base of the bladder (the trigone) and obstructed the ureters, the tubes that connect the kidneys to the bladder.

Because prostate cancer symptoms are nonspecific, and because they resemble symptoms of benign prostate conditions, the only way to find out is through thorough screening with tests that will eliminate all other possibilities.

Metastatic Cancer

The spread of cancer from the prostate to other areas of the body is called metastasis, which can happen three ways: through the lymphatic system (lymph nodes and fluids), the vascular system (blood vessels), or extracapsular extension. For example, the tumor could break through the prostate wall and invade the fat surrounding the gland, or move into the neurovascular bundles. Because cells take the path of least resistance to get out, the neurovascular bundles are often the target. The potential for metastasis depends on volume of the tumor and aggressiveness of the cancer cells. Larger-volume tumors are more likely to metastasize, and so are tumors with poorly differentiated or aggressive cells.

When cells break away from a tumor, they find other hosts and new colonies form. The apex of the prostate, where it is joined to the urethra, is the most common place for cancer to break through. Other sites of local metastasis are usually the lymph nodes and seminal vesicles. When traveling farther, it is more common for prostate cancer cells to go directly to the skeletal system. The cancer can travel to other organs including the liver or the lung. Metastasis of prostate cancer to the brain is not as common.

Cancer is always identified by the primary site.

Symptoms of Metastatic Prostate Cancer

Because prostate cancer rarely causes symptoms in the early stage, men often do not become aware of the disease until they have symptoms of distant spread. Persistent and often severe bone pain in the back or hip is a common symptom of metastatic cancer. The most common site of metastasis—about 70 percent—is the spine, but cancer also travels to the ribs, pelvis, femur, and shoulder.

The pelvic lymph nodes are another common site of metastatic cancer, often swelling and obstructing the flow of lymph fluid. Such swelling, called lymphedema, occurs in the legs, feet, and scrotum. The presence of these symptoms should be studied with a bone scan and CAT (computerized axial tomography) scan to determine the extent of metastasis.

Urinary symptoms are very much like those of BPH. There may be more urgency to urinate, more frequent urination, a burning sensation, or blood in the urine. There could also be blood in the semen and a decrease in the amount of semen ejaculated. By themselves, these are not symptoms of cancer, but they suggest that the urethra or ejaculatory ducts are blocked by something. When cancer is advanced, it may cause impotence or a less rigid erection.

Hormone-Refractory Prostate Cancer

Symptoms of prostate cancer can be controlled by depriving the body of male hormones. Hormone-refractory prostate cancer no longer responds to treatment with these hormones. All prostate cancer eventually becomes resistant to hormonal manipulation for reasons still not clearly understood. The length of time it takes to reach this point is different in all men, and new ways of applying hormone treatment have helped to delay this process. Although prostate cancer does not respond to traditional chemotherapy, it is sometimes used to treat hormone-refractory prostate cancer.

4

Understanding the Risk Factors

$\mathbf{W}$e do not yet know the cause of prostate cancer, but we do know the strongest risk factor is age, despite the recent discovery of a prostate cancer gene implicating family history as a risk factor for so-called hereditary prostate cancer. Cancer of any kind can be defined as an acquired genetic disease produced by exposure to environmental carcinogens that have caused damage to normal cells over the course of years. During our lifetime, we are all exposed to potential carcinogens in the environment– cigarettes, radiation, gasoline, animal fats, pesticides. The development of prostate cancer is a multistage process and the passage of time is needed for these chance exposures to accumulate and produce the mutations in our genes that cause the cancer.

In the United States, where one in four deaths is from cancer, men have a 50 percent lifetime risk of developing prostate cancer by the time they are 80. Lifetime risk is the probability that anyone over the course of a lifetime will develop cancer or die from it. However, the relative risk must also be taken into consideration. This risk is a measure of the relationship between risk factors and a particular cancer. Relative risk increases with exposure to a particular environmental element, or there is an inherited predisposition. Smokers, for example, have 10 times the relative risk of developing lung cancer compared with nonsmokers. A woman with a mother or sister with breast cancer has a far greater risk of developing that cancer.

Aging

The longer you live, the greater the risk of prostate cancer. More than 80 percent of prostate cancers are found in men over 65, and more than 90 percent of deaths are in this age group. Many autopsy studies have revealed that men who died of other causes had prostate cancer so microscopic it had never been discovered. About 20 percent of men in their 50s are believed to have microscopic, latent cancer cells that may or may not clinically manifest or become symptomatic in their lifetime. But we are beginning to realize that younger men–3 out of 10 men in their 30s and 40s–have potentially precancerous cells in their prostates known as prostatic intraepithelial neoplasia (PIN). PIN is not yet a cancer, but high-grade PIN is potentially a precursor to cancer. (See Chapter 2.)

By age 40, the chances accelerate of getting prostate cancer, doubling every decade until about age 80. For the majority–about 70 percent–of patients diagnosed with prostate cancer, the only risk factor they have is their advancing age.

Family History

If your father had prostate cancer, your risk is about double that of a man whose father did not have the disease. The risk increases with the number of family members. For example, if your father and grandfather, or your father and brother have it, you are 5 times more likely to get it. If three men in your family have it, such as your father, grandfather, and a brother or uncle, the risk increases to 11 times.

Until the discovery of the prostate cancer gene in 1996, there was no conclusive link between family history and incidence of prostate cancer. That is, we were not sure if the family connection was genetic or environmental, the idea being that people in the same families may experience the same environmental or dietary risk factors.

When this gene–HPC1 for hereditary prostate cancer–is inherited in mutated form, it predisposes a man to prostate cancer. The risk of developing prostate cancer by age 80 is about 50 percent in all men, but if you have the mutated gene the risk increases to 88 percent.

Although this discovery is important, it accounts for only a small number—perhaps 3 percent—of prostate cancers. Men who get prostate cancer early in life are thought to carry this gene, just as women with the BRCA1 breast cancer gene get breast cancer earlier than most women. The discovery of the prostate cancer gene may also shed some light on genetic factors responsible for the high incidence of this cancer in African American men.

When prostate cancer occurs in several members of a family, it is likely to be a more aggressive form of the cancer, and thus it appears at an earlier age. Most urologists believe men with a history of this cancer on their father's—or their mother's—side of the family should begin screening no later than age 40. (See Chapters 5 and 6.)

There has been some speculation that if your mother has breast cancer, you are at increased risk for prostate cancer. More research must be done, however, before we can be certain of this connection.

Race

African American men have the highest rate of prostate cancer in the world, and native Chinese and Japanese men have among the lowest rate. The incidence of prostate cancer is low in Chinese men until they move to the United States, suggesting lifestyle has some effect. Is it the dietary switch from fish and rice to bacon cheeseburgers? Whether or not geography and diet are important risk factors for prostate cancer remains to be proven.

When we look at a racial and ethnic cross section of men at age 50, latent prostate cancer in all men is equal; there are no interracial variations. About 20 percent of these men will have latent prostate cancer among all races. The potential interracial differences come with the rate of progression of the disease, which may be influenced by genetics and diet.

African American men generally discover prostate cancer later, which could be why the death rate is double that of white men, but it does not mean the cancer is more aggressive. It could mean that these men as a group have less access to quality health care or they are less likely to participate in early detection programs.

We need to do more research to compare the PSA levels in similar communities. For example, is the PSA rate affected by the size or density of the prostate? Or by the amount of testosterone produced? So far, much of the research into prostate cancer has compared apples to oranges rather than apples to apples. PSA rates should be compared among men with the same racial background, age, and prostate size. This is being done in the Chinese community in New York City. In exchange for free screenings, these men have become part of a large study on prostate cancer. Each year the men are invited back to repeat the test, so that the PSA results can be monitored over a period of years.

One of the areas of investigation is the difference in the PSA levels in Chinese and non-Chinese men. A 4.0 PSA is considered normal for a white man from North America or Europe, but should it be the same for a Chinese man with a smaller prostate? Perhaps the PSA level must be measured against the size or density of the prostate. The density of the PSA may be higher in a smaller prostate. Chapter 6 includes comparisons of PSA levels in African Americans, Asians, and white men.

Environment and Diet

Many variables affect the growth of cancer cells, from genetic susceptibility to diet to exposure to carcinogens. Perhaps something in our environment—in the industrialized western world—causes prostate cells to become cancerous. Interestingly, the dog is the only animal that gets prostate cancer. Is this because the dog lives in our environment?

Studies have highlighted certain occupational risks. For example, higher death rates from prostate cancer are reported in farmers, mechanics, welders, plumbers, newspaper workers, and men who work with metals or rubber manufacturing. No occupation has been linked conclusively, but some research suggests that men exposed to cadmium—welders and electroplate workers—may be at increased risk. Cadmium is a trace mineral found in cigarette smoke and alkaline batteries. It is related indirectly because it diffuses the body's zinc, which is necessary for cellular growth. Of all body organs, the prostate has the highest need for zinc.

In these studies we cannot be sure if these men are at greater risk because of their jobs, or because they might be eating higher-fat diets, or perhaps they smoke more than other men. Much more research is necessary.

A change of diet is not as dramatically therapeutic against prostate cancer as quitting smoking would be in preventing lung cancer, but you are more likely to have many other health problems if your diet is loaded with animal fats and no fiber from grains, vegetables, and fruits.

High-Animal-Fat Diet

We know that too much animal fat clogs the arteries and this increases the risk of heart attack, but does a high-fat diet also cause prostate cancer? Many medical scientists believe it does, but all the evidence is not in yet. Animal fat or protein, such as that found in meat and butter, is said to be more harmful than vegetable fats such as olive oil and certain fish oils. There tends to be less prostate cancer in regions where fish is a big part of the diet. Also, supplements of marine fish oils were shown in some studies to lower the risk, because some fish oil is believed to contain other fats that protect against cancer.

Animal fat, especially red meat, has been heavily implicated in prostate cancer. Although we do not know if a high-fat diet causes prostate cancer, we know that there is some evidence in animal studies to suggest that it may affect the course of the disease. Conversely, these studies also suggest that a low-fat diet can often be considered a way to slow the progression of prostate cancer.

A Harvard study showed a 79 percent increase in risk for men who eat a high-fat diet. One theory is that dietary fat increases the serum sex hormone levels. A study showed that when fat consumption was lowered, these hormone levels in the urine were lower, too. Studies also show that diet is most strongly related to risk, so change can be beneficial.

Earlier studies at Harvard have proven to medical investigators that men who eat a lot of fat, at least five or more servings a week of red meat, for example, are at the highest risk for prostate cancer. Their risk is almost double that of men who do not eat this much. Researchers theorize that this increase may be because fat is necessary for the production of testosterone, which in turn feeds the prostate cancer cells. Fat contains an ingredient called alpha-linolenic acid, which is found in red meat, whole milk, butter, and processed soybean oil. Some investigators believe it is an active agent in promoting prostate cancer.

Studies at Memorial Sloan-Kettering Cancer Center found that prostate tumors implanted in mice grew only half as fast in those with diets of about 21 percent fat compared with diets of about 40 percent fat, which is what most American men consume. Tumors did not disappear, but the slower growth rate was impressive. Most prostate cancers develop around the age of 60, so if you change your diet to slow down the growth, you may live many more years without clinical progression of the cancer. Interestingly, tumor growth was two and a half times greater in mice fed the high-fat diet.

A new dietary study of men who have prostate cancer was begun by Dr. William Fair, chief of urology, and his colleague, Dr. Warren Heston, at Memorial Sloan-Kettering Cancer Center, in collaboration with the American Health Foundation. Half the men are consuming a normal diet with 30 percent of their calories coming from fat. The other half are consuming only 15 percent of their calories from fat.

This research is being done to find out why there are such vast differences in the incidence of prostate cancer in the United States. Autopsies have shown that the incidence of undiagnosed latent prostate cancer is about the same in American men as in Chinese men, but the incidence of full-blown clinical cancer is 120 times greater in the United States than it is in China, where men eat a low-fat, high-fiber diet.

Although there is meat in the Chinese diet, there is less of it, because the bulk of a meal is made up of grains and vegetables. In the United States, meat often provides more than half the calories for a meal. When compared with the Chinese, Americans eat 6 times more meat and eggs, 55 times more milk, slightly more fats and oils, and 3 times more fruit than the Chinese. The Chinese, on the other hand, eat 3 times more fish and grain and 30 times more vegetables. Overall, the American diet contains 43 percent fat, whereas the Chinese diet contains less than 20 percent.

Much research has been done and continues to be done about the effect of what we eat on our risk of cancer. Although no nutrients have been proven to prevent cancer, many scientists believe a low-fat diet can slow the growth of already slow-growing prostate cancer. While we cannot say that a man who eats lots of animal fat and no fiber will get prostate cancer, neither can we say for sure that every person who smokes will get lung cancer. However, the odds are stacked against high-fat consumers and smokers. Most lung cancer is found among smokers. Most prostate cancer is found in societies with high-animal-fat and high-animal-protein diets. Studies tell us that Western populations, where red meat is highly consumed, have more cancer–prostate, breast, and colon–than communities where it is not, such as Asia. Additionally, the highest number of overweight people live in the industrialized nations.

If research is correct and too much animal fat has an effect on prostate cancer, then by changing your diet you can quite possibly slow down its development. Very few American men who have had treatment for prostate cancer ask if they should change their diet to make themselves healthier, yet most Chinese patients ask.

Vegetables and Fruit

Vegetables and fruit are not only good sources of fiber and vitamins, but they may contain other elements that play a role in cancer prevention. Chemists analyzing vegetables have discovered some compounds that seem to retard the cell breakdowns that result in cancer. The scientific community has only just begun to study our diets and there are many things they don't know. There could be elements in vegetables that *give* us cancer, too, although the positive benefits appear to far outweigh any potential hazards.

Pesticides and fertilizers are also under scrutiny by medical researchers. The metabolic fate of toxic chemicals synthesized by plants as a defense against bugs, animals, and bacteria is extremely complex and varies greatly in every individual.

Variety and moderation offer the best protection from the carcinogens we cannot avoid, whether they are pesticides used to grow our fruits and vegetables, hormones fed to market animals, or pollutants ingested by fish. If we tried to avoid everything that might potentially cause a cell mutation, we would starve to death.

•   **Tomatoes.**   A 9-year study of 47,000 men showed that 10 servings a week of tomato-based foods reduce the risk of prostate cancer by 20 percent. According to a Harvard University study by Dr. Edward Giovannucci reported in *The Journal of the National Cancer Institute,* more was better, and in any form–juice, sauce, raw, or on pizza. Spaghetti sauce was the most common "tomato" food eaten by the men. Tomatoes are rich in an antioxidant called lycopene, which makes them one of the few vegetables that are more beneficial cooked than raw. Apparently heat makes the cells burst and release more lycopene. (See "Antioxidants" below.)

• **Soy.** Several studies have concentrated on soy products, including one at the comprehensive cancer center at the University of Alabama, to find out if the consumption of soy foods reduces the risk of prostate cancer. Genisten is an element found in soybeans and some cruciferous vegetables, which blocks angiogenesis—the growth of new blood vessels. If genisten could be used in treatment, it might prevent cancer cells from developing new capillaries that supply blood to tumors.

• **Antioxidants.** Certain foods contain antioxidants, which act like our body's own nutrition police, protecting us from free radicals. While we are breathing and burning up energy, our cells continuously generate hazardous waste that can set the stage for cancer. This waste is made of molecules known as free radicals. Poor nutrition leaves our antioxidant levels low. Vitamins A, C, and E are all antioxidants. Good food sources are melons and citrus fruits, yellow and green vegetables, tomatoes, green leafy vegetables, potatoes, wheat germ, oatmeal, peanuts, and brown rice. Garlic and broccoli are especially rich in antioxidants. In fact, the National Cancer Institute puts garlic high on its list of natural antioxidants. Eaten raw, garlic also stimulates immunological functions, lowers blood cholesterol, thins blood, and helps prevent embolisms.

Cruciferous vegetables such as broccoli, cabbage, cauliflower, and brussels sprouts contain substances that are thought to inhibit cancer in animals, but there is still no definitive proof that they protect humans.

Vitamins C and E may have preventive components according to some studies. However, large numbers of people must be studied for long periods of time before we can come to any conclusions about the benefit of vitamins in preventing cancer. A well-balanced diet provides most of the vitamins we need.

Unproved Risk Factors

• **The Sunbelt Theory.** Because prostate cancer rates are highest in the northeastern part of the United States and lowest in the Sunbelt, a connection has been made between exposure to vitamin D—the sunshine vitamin—and prostate cancer. Sunlight stimulates the body to make vitamin D. It is thought this vitamin inhibits the growth of tumors, that it somehow prevents microscopic prostate tumors from progressing. Only small amounts of sun exposure are needed to produce vitamin D. This vitamin can also be ingested with fish or fortified milk. Although this theory has not been proven yet, the idea is plausible and studies continue.

• **Benign Prostate Conditions.** BPH has symptoms similar to prostate cancer and both diseases depend on hormonal stimulation from testosterone. Both develop as a man ages, and BPH can coexist with cancer, but no direct link has been found.

• **Vasectomy.** For a while there was suspicion that men who had vesectomies were at higher risk for developing prostate cancer, but this suspicion is unfounded. The increased incidence of prostate cancer is believed to be due to a selection bias. Men who undergo vasectomy have it performed by a urologist and are thus more likely to have follow-up with their urologist for prostate cancer screening or if new voiding symptoms develop. Thus, they are more likely to discover prostate cancer.

PART TWO

Guidelines for Diagnosis and Staging

5

Diagnostic Tests

The symptoms of prostate cancer are not always brought to medical attention until the cancer has grown large within the prostate or spread outside the prostate. Regular screening is a potentially lifesaving procedure. The two basic screening tools for early detection are the digital rectal exam (DRE) and a prostate-specific antigen (PSA) blood test. Both of these simple tests can be done in a doctor's office.

Because the PSA blood test is an easy way to screen for prostate cancer, this test is sometimes substituted by the internist or family doctor for a DRE, but this is unfortunate because the PSA alone is not always accurate. The next chapter is devoted to the variables of the PSA.

Digital Rectal Examination (DRE)

Because the prostate is located near the anal opening, most of the back wall of the gland can be reached and palpated by the doctor's gloved finger. By pushing the finger forward toward the pubic bone, the doctor can tell if the normally smooth surface of the prostate feels abnormal, if it is enlarged, or if there are any lumps or bumps. A tumor or cancerous lesion often begins as a small, hard nodule. The back wall–the peripheral zone–is where about 70 percent of the cancers occur.

The American Cancer Society and the National Cancer Institute recommend an annual DRE and PSA test as a screening tool for prostate cancer for every man over the age of 50. The American Urological Association suggests an annual DRE and PSA beginning at age 40 if anyone in the family had prostate cancer, and for all men between 50 and 70. This group also urges African American men, who have double the death rate from prostate cancer of white men, to begin screening at age 40.

The DRE can detect about half the prostate cancers, but alone it is not enough. Most lumps and bumps turn out not to be cancer. Some nodules will actually turn out to be stones, scarifications from previous surgery, BPH, or inflammatory lesions. A nodule felt on DRE has a 50 percent chance on biopsy of being cancerous.

The size of the prostate is also significant in understanding the effectiveness of the DRE. In Asians the prostate is smaller, and in African American men it is larger, which can mean that more or less of the gland itself is available for inspection.

If the prostate is enlarged because of BPH or any other condition, a small nodule of cancer lurking in the area could be missed. It is also difficult to detect tumors that are deep inside the prostate.

Prior to widespread use of PSA for the early detection of prostate cancer, DRE alone was the only way it was found, usually during an annual physical exam. BPH, prostatitis, prostatic calculi, infarction, or postsurgical or biopsy changes must be included in the differential diagnosis of an abnormal DRE.

The DRE characteristically underestimates tumor volume and the extent of progression as the intragland mass is usually greater than the digitally identified cancer. Extracapsular spread of cancer is identified in 40 to 60 percent of prostate specimens after radical prostatectomy in patients who are believed to have clinically localized cancer before surgery. This is called understaging.

Many biologically significant cancers are not associated with signs and symptoms, and limitations of DRE are evident when considering that over half the prostate cancers that are believed before surgery to be clinically localized have evidence of extension when examined by the pathologist after radical surgery. The limits of the DRE are further highlighted by results of PSA screening. Combining PSA and DRE provides more effective direction of early prostate cancer than either test alone.

In addition to size, the DRE can also pick up any nodules or areas of asymmetry or firmness that may be suspicious for prostate cancer. It must be emphasized that size of prostate alone is not an accurate predictor nor is it correlated to degree of symptoms and outcome after treatment. If a nodule or firmness is found on DRE, a referral to a urologist is appropriate so that a transrectal ultrasound and possible needle biopsy of the nodule can be performed.

If the DRE and PSA are both normal, there is probably no cancer present. If the DRE is normal but the PSA is high, then further tests should be done to rule out cancer.

Clinical Biopsy

Prostate ultrasonography is the next step in trying to diagnose prostate cancer after the physical exam and PSA. Ultrasound is like radar. Sound waves bouncing from the prostate become images on a screen. This is a diagnostic tool to look at the prostate and the area around it. It also guides the physician's needle in removing samples of prostate tissue for biopsy.

The biopsy determines whether or not there are cancer cells in the prostate, how aggressive they are, and approximately where they are. It does not necessarily tell us how far the cancer might have spread. That is determined by a pathological examination of tissue removed during surgery or as a result of diagnostic scans such as computerized tomography (CT) and bone scans. If surgery is performed to remove the gland, then the prostate itself is analyzed, the surrounding organs examined, and the pelvic lymph nodes removed for pathological examination.

Transrectal Ultrasound (TRUS)

Until 1988, the only way we could look at the prostate was to insert a long needle blindly through the rectum. Now, with more sophisticated imaging techniques and the PSA, we have been able to learn a great deal more about the prostate. By inserting an ultrasound probe into the rectum, the physician can scan the prostate. The sonogram can also be used to measure prostate volume or size to gauge the degree of enlargement and to see any suspicious lesions.

The clinical biopsy is usually performed in the urologist's office during the transrectal ultrasound (TRUS) procedure and is one of the easiest cancer biopsies. A long needle is inserted through the TRUS probe into the prostate to draw out some cells. Tissue samples are usually taken from six different areas of the prostate (in addition to areas that look suspicious) to obtain the most accurate possible reading of cellular activity. This reading is known as a sextant biopsy. More than six samples may be taken in a particularly large prostate. (Prostate tissue from the transition zone can also be analyzed when it is removed from the inner core with a resectoscope as part of the transurethral resection of the prostate procedure, explained in Chapter 2.)

The TRUS procedure takes advance planning. Aspirin products must be avoided for 7 days prior to the exam to prevent excess bleeding after the biopsy. Two to three hours before the exam, a patient gives himself a Fleet enema to empty out the rectum. The physician will also prescribe an antibiotic to prevent rectal bacteria from being carried into the prostate by the needle. The needle biopsy could also spread bacteria to a heart valve or prosthetic joint. Men who have a liver condition such as cirrhosis, or who are taking blood thinners such as warfarin (Coumadin), may need to take other precautions. A primary care physician should be consulted before the biopsy is done in these cases.

The procedure itself is simple. The patient lies on the exam table on his side, bringing his knees up to his chest. The TRUS probe is covered with a condom and inserted into the anus. The long needle that will take samples of prostate tissue is inserted inside the probe. Although there is not much pain, there is some pressure and a pinch. When the doctor releases the needle from the probe, it sounds like a staple gun. It is the anticipation of the "bang" of the spring-loaded biopsy gun that unnerves many men. Most doctors talk with their patients to relax them so that they are not taken by surprise.

Six tissue samples must be taken: from the front, middle, and back portions of the right and left lobes of the prostate. Still, with such a small needle, a cancer can be overlooked. There is a 35 percent margin for error that the needle will miss the cancer. By taking samples from six sites, these odds are minimized. This method is not foolproof, but the biopsy results must be considered with all of the other diagnostic tests.

Although the physician is watching the video monitor during this procedure to serve as a guide for the needle shots, he or she will not generally say what is on the screen. The tissue is sent to the lab and a report usually takes about a week. The video monitor also scans the bladder, ejaculatory duct, and seminal vesicles for signs of cancer.

Risks of side effects from this type of biopsy are minimal. Following the procedure, there may be blood in the urine or stool for 3 to 4 days and blood in the semen for a month or more. Your doctor will probably prescribe oral antibiotics for a period of time and recommend abstention from sex for a week. Infection or serious bleeding is rare, but if bleeding is continuous or heavy, consult your doctor.

Transurethral Resection of the Prostate (TURP)

This procedure is primarily used to remove tissue from inside the prostate (around the doughnut hole) to relieve pressure on the urethra when the prostate becomes so enlarged that it squeezes the urethra and makes it difficult to urinate. However, it may also be used as a method to biopsy tissue at the inner core of the prostate.

A fiberoptic telescope is inserted through the penis via the urethra. Through this tube the urologist can see and use an electric loop to remove and cauterize prostate tissue. (See Chapter 2 for more information about this procedure.)

Other Staging Tests

Staging for prostate cancer is done in two phases. The first is the clinical stage, which is based on all the diagnostic tests that can be done without surgery. This clinical staging is generally able to determine the aggressiveness of the cancer. The pathological staging is determined after surgery when the prostate itself as well as the lymph nodes indicate whether or not the cancer has extended out of the capsule of the prostate or has metastasized to the lymph nodes or other organs.

Naturally, if you do not have surgery, your treatment will be determined by your clinical biopsy and the results of staging tests such as bone and CAT scans. There is more information about staging in Chapter 7. In addition to the diagnostic procedures already described, there are others that may give us more information without the need for surgery.

Bone Scan

Because prostate cancer often metastasizes to the bones before it goes to other organs, a bone scan is often included as part of the diagnostic workup, especially if you have a high PSA. A bone scan is a radioactive isotope scan of the skeletal system.

A bone scan is usually done on an outpatient basis in a nuclear medicine facility in a hospital or a radiologist's office. After a radioactive isotope is injected into the veins, the entire body is scanned. The isotope makes bones appear in the picture so that any abnormalities show up as "hot spots." The test is painless and the isotope used for the pictures is eventually washed out of the body. It poses no harm or risk to the patient or anyone who is in contact with him.

Hot spots are suspected metastases, but they could also be due to arthritis, previously broken bones, or other injuries, so the test is not totally accurate. If hot spots show up in the bone scan, then more tests are required to get more details.

Because studies show that the likelihood of a positive bone scan in patients with PSAs less than 10 is low, many urologists no longer order bone scans in patients with a PSA less than this level because it is not cost-effective.

Computerized Axial Tomography (CAT) Scan

A CAT scan–computerized axial tomography–is an excellent way to look at the lymph node–bearing areas of the lower abdomen, liver, and other solid organs for signs of metastasis. Not all physicians order this test because of the expense and the low likelihood of finding significant tumor activity. However, many urologists feel it is better to have the test performed before making a treatment decision.

The test is painless and not uncomfortable. The patient lies inside a wide tube and the X-ray camera rotates around the body and translates information into two-dimensional "slices" or cross sections. The radiation dose from a CAT scan is considerably higher than a routine X-ray. The amount depends on the number of slices needed to get an accurate picture. CAT is also used in planning radiation treatment to outline the field or area to be treated.

Magnetic Resonance Imaging (MRI)

Magnetic resonance imaging (MRI) is sometimes used to verify images of a bone scan. MRI is like a giant magnet that measures magnetic energy from the cells. Like a CAT scan, it can give a better image of the solid organs and lymph nodes. Scientists are developing the MRI capability to differentiate between malignant and benign processes and to evaluate lymph nodes for metastasis. Patients are often anxious about the procedure because it means being confined in a long, noisy, and narrow tube for as long as an hour. However, a mild sedative makes most claustrophobic patients relax. Open-air MRI is becoming available at some diagnostic centers.

ProstaScint Scan

In 1996, the FDA approved the ProstaScint scan for use in the staging of prostate cancer. Developed by the Cytogen Corporation, this scan utilizes monoclonal antibodies that are attached to a radioactive isotope. The monoclonal antibodies are directed against prostate-specific membrane antigens (PSMAs) found on the surface of prostate cancer cells. If prostate cancer is present, the monoclonal antibodies attach themselves to it and the radioactive isotope scan can detect its location.

The ProstaScint may therefore detect the extent of prostate cancer prior to therapy and the location of disease recurrence after treatment.

The Cost of Screening

Some of the routine costs of screening are minimal. These are normally included as part of routine annual physical examinations in the doctor's office, such as the DRE. The PSA blood sample is evaluated by a laboratory, however, so there are additional costs. Some medical insurance plans may not cover this cost if you are under a certain age or if you have a PSA done more than once a year.

The TRUS procedure can cost as much as $900 for the combined sonogram and biopsy. In addition, laboratory fees for pathology can run more than $50 per core sample. A sextant biopsy costs $300. A bone scan or CAT scan can cost from $600 to $1,500. Such testing is often available at clinics where the cost for a TRUS procedure could be as low as $100.

Ask what other charges to expect and call your insurance company to be sure you know what is covered. The DRE, PSA, and TRUS are covered by Medicaid, Medicare, and most health insurance plans, although they may have caps on how much will be paid.

If you are uninsured, call your local chapter of the American Cancer Society or the National Cancer Institute. Local hospitals, physicians, and health organizations sometimes offer reduced cost screenings, especially during Prostate Cancer Awareness Week. There may also be free screening in your neighborhood similar to a clinic in New York City's Chinatown, which offers free screenings to the community for 1 or 2 weeks every year. Men over 50 can get free DREs and PSAs while a cooperating laboratory provides the pathological evaluation free of charge.

Questions to Ask About Screening

If you are in the hands of a certified urologist, that physician will do most of the screening. But screening can be done at diagnostic centers, in hospital outpatient departments, and sometimes in the office of a primary care physician. Standards may vary from facility to facility. Before you go for a screening, ask what exactly will be done and who will do it. There are certain screening standards.

- **What will be the urologist's role in the screening?**
While there may be technicians present during testing, the urologist is in charge and should always be present.

- **What will the tests determine?**
Diagnostic tests are important because they help to determine exactly where the cancer is, how big it is, and how aggressive it is. Because symptoms could be caused by many things other than cancer, such tests are critical to rule out other disease.

- **Will more tests be necessary?**
As we have explained in this chapter, each test brings the diagnosis to a new level. For example, the DRE and PSA may indicate that you have prostate cancer, then a biopsy becomes necessary, and if that indicates the presence of cancer, then more tests will be needed to determine if it has spread.

- **Am I receiving all the tests I need for the best diagnosis?**
Some insurance plans will not cover more than one test, and some

physicians also do not use additional tests if they believe the odds are slim that metastasis will be found. Always ask for an explanation, and if you believe you need the additional tests, talk with your physician and your health insurer to find a way to have the test.

- **Who will perform the tests–a physician, technician, or nurse?**

While a DRE would only be done by your primary care physician or urologist, the blood taken for the PSA would most likely be taken by a technician, nurse, or physician's assistant. More complex tests requiring sophisticated equipment, or that are more invasive, are usually done by physicians and technicians.

- **Will there be any side effects to the tests?**

Some tests, such as the TRUS, may have mild side effects such as blood in the urine, semen, and stool. Also, there might be a burning sensation when urinating, as well as frequency and urgency, for a while after the procedure.

- **Where and by whom will the prostate tissue be examined?**

Ask about the pathologist and the pathology laboratory. Find out if the pathology will be done in the same medical center or in another laboratory. You might check with your insurance company to make sure it covers the particular pathology laboratory.

- **How long will it take to learn the results of the clinical biopsy?**

It should take 4 to 6 business days to find out the results. Ask your doctor for an estimated time to call for results. Understand that if this takes longer, it does not necessarily mean the results are bad; it only means your anxiety level is higher. Sometimes there are delays in hospitals and laboratories.

6

The Controversial PSA Test

This simple blood test has revolutionized screening for prostate cancer and heralded an increase in the number of men who are diagnosed with prostate cancer that is potentially curable because of early detection. The PSA blood test is a tumor marker that measures levels of a protein called prostate-specific antigen in the blood. The test was approved by the Food and Drug Administration (FDA) in 1994 for the early detection of prostate cancer provided it is used in combination with the digital rectal examination (DRE).

PSA is a type of protein molecule, known as serine protease, produced by the epithelial cells of the prostate. The purpose of PSA is to liquefy the gelatinous seminal fluid once it is inside the female reproductive tract. PSA is normally present in the blood of all men in low amounts. When PSA is elevated, a "process" is disrupting the normal ductal architecture of the prostate, causing more PSA to leak into the blood. This leaking can be caused by benign prostate disease such as BPH, infections such as prostatitis, as well as prostate cancer, so the PSA test alone cannot determine the presence of cancer.

For example, the PSA rises with BPH, but usually not as fast as it does with prostate cancer. However, the PSA reading could be confused if the prostate is enlarged with BPH and cancer is also present. The two most definitely can coexist. To add to the confusion, a man who is taking finasteride (Proscar) to treat BPH would have a reduced PSA level. It could decrease to half the normal baseline value. PSA levels also increase after ejaculation, so having a blood test for PSA within 24 hours of ejaculation could present a falsely high reading. The same thing can happen after riding a bicycle for any length of time where the pressure of the bicycle seat may irritate the prostate gland.

PSA levels can go into the hundreds or thousands in cases of acute prostatitis or if a recent needle biopsy has been performed on the prostate. A high reading generally means something may be wrong and investigation with ultrasound or biopsy should be considered. However, it does not automatically mean prostate cancer is present. Many men who show PSA levels of 10 and higher do not have cancer.

How PSA Is Measured

Because PSA is produced by the prostate gland and not the prostate cancer, it is a prostate-specific substance, not a cancer-specific substance. Therein lies the controversy. It is possible to have prostate cancer and still have a normal PSA. Some men—about 40 percent—with prostate cancer have PSA levels under 4. Moreover, 25 percent of men with BPH have PSA levels higher than 4. Taken together, the usefulness of the PSA alone is limited in the early detection of potentially curable prostate cancer. It is difficult to tell the difference between cancer and BPH when the PSA level is between 4 and 10.

Now, here is another aspect to add to the dilemma. PSA exists in more than one molecular form in the blood. From 60 to 95 percent of PSA in the blood is bound to another substance—alpha$_1$ antichymotrypsin—while most of the rest is circulating free and unbound. Studies suggest that prostate cancer detection is more accurate if we analyze the ratio of the free unbound PSA with the total PSA. Detection ability may improve as much as 20 percent.

The PSA is measured in nanograms per milliliter (ng/mL) of blood serum. The normal range is 0.1 to 4.0 ng/mL. The assay used for measuring PSA does not go to zero, so the lowest possible measure is 0.1, and this may vary for each laboratory. (For purposes of simplicity, the ng/mL is omitted in the text and only the numbers are used.) While the laboratory baseline reading for a normal PSA is less than 4.0, this level has a different meaning for a 40-year-old and an 80-year-old. For men over 70, for instance, a 6.5 is considered normal.

Adjusting for Age and Race

PSA's usefulness as a tumor marker depends on proper variables of age and race. PSA is produced by the epithelial cells that line ducts of the prostate gland. It is well known that the prostate gland increases in size with age. In general, older men have more tissue to produce PSA and therefore a greater likelihood that PSA will leak into the blood, since the normal barriers that keep PSA in the ductal system are less tight because BPH and sometimes inflammation have disrupted the internal architecture of the prostate gland.

It is no longer appropriate to use one reference range for men of all ages. Investigators have shown that the use of age-specific ranges makes the PSA more sensitive in younger men and more specific in older men. These ranges also improve detection of curable cancer in younger men and the decision not to do invasive biopsies in older men.

Asians have smaller prostates compared to Caucasians of the same age. African Americans have more prostate cancer. Several studies of the distribution of PSA levels have been done by Dr. Joseph Oesterling of the University of Michigan, and age-specific guidelines have been established for white, African American, and Japanese men:

Normal Age-Specific Reference Ranges
(PSA values in ng/mL)

Age	Japanese	African Americans	Caucasians
40 to 49	0 to 2.0	0 to 2.0	0 to 2.5
50 to 59	0 to 3.0	0 to 4.0	0 to 3.5
60 to 69	0 to 4.0	0 to 4.5	0 to 4.5
70 to 79	0 to 5.0	0 to 5.5	0 to 6.5

By using narrower reference ranges, the sensitivity of PSA as a tumor marker is increased, which should help in the early detection of cancers in younger men in their 40s or 50s. By using wider reference ranges in men 60 and over, the specificity of the test is increased, which means that many men in their 60s and 70s are spared further invasive testing, for example, with ultrasound needle biopsy. However, it could also mean that some of the older men would not have their cancer detected.

With these age-specific reference ranges, we can develop a more accurate diagnostic picture for early curable prostate cancer.

- If the PSA is within the normal range and the DRE is not remarkable, the patient should be followed with annual checkups to monitor for change.
- If the PSA level is greater than the age-specific range and the DRE is unremarkable, an ultrasound biopsy should be done.
- If the DRE is abnormal in spite of a normal PSA, then an ultrasound biopsy should be done.

Adjusting for Density and Velocity

There are three factors that influence PSA levels in men with prostate cancer: the volume of cancer, the volume of BPH, and the grade of cancer. The variable that correlates most closely with PSA is the cancer volume.

There is a variable amount of BPH tissue in men with and without prostate cancer that contributes to the overall PSA. Thus, PSA values appear to overlap greatly in men with prostate cancers of similar stage and between men with glands that harbor cancer cells and BPH. Another complication is that on a volume-to-volume basis, poorly differentiated cancers produce less PSA than do well-differentiated cancers.

PSA is not a perfect marker. It has confounding variables. Two methods of coping with these variables are to look at the PSA density (PSA-D) and velocity (PSA-V). Density is the ratio of PSA compared to the size, or volume, of the prostate. Velocity is the rate of increase of PSA. Density can be measured with ultrasound biopsy and velocity can be measured with periodic blood tests.

In general, cancer raises PSA levels more than BPH. Since PSA is related to the volume of cancer, it seems reasonable that men with cancer should have a more rapid rise in PSA. We have evidence that there are significant differences in rate of change in PSA in men with cancer and those with BPH. One way to distinguish between the two is to use the average PSA velocity. This is determined by measuring PSA three times at least six months apart over a 2-year period. Velocity may be best used to follow men with normal PSA levels and those who have had a biopsy with no evidence of cancer.

Screening Dilemmas

Although some studies suggest that the PSA test could find 80 percent of aggressive prostate cancers 5 to 10 years before they are clinically evident, there is also a 35 percent margin for error in this test. Forty percent of men who have known prostate cancer have a PSA within normal limits. If a PSA level is high, all other reasons for this elevation must be ruled out before the physician can determine if the cause is cancer. In order to rule out cancer, you will likely need a biopsy.

By screening with PSA, about 20 percent of the cancers found are clinically indolent, which is the root of the controversy about whether it is helpful or harmful for a man to know he has this cancer. Prostate cancer is the only cancer with such a high disparity between the occult—latent—and the clinical. Clearly, screening for prostate cancer is not useful unless it helps people live longer.

When men first come to their doctors with prostate cancer, about one third have potentially curable cancers, whereas the other two thirds have cancer that has already broken through the wall of the prostate or has metastasized. Among those with potentially curable cancer who choose surgery, about half will have their cancer upstaged after surgery when more information is available from the pathologist who has examined the prostate and surrounding tissue. About a third of this group may develop local or metastasized cancer 10 years after radical prostatectomy.

So what is the value of aggressive therapy? Now that the PSA has allowed us to detect latent cancer in large populations, there are many controversies about treatment. There is an argument that identifying a large population of men offers nothing if curative therapy is not available.

Before the survival benefits of universal early screening can be endorsed, we need more studies. We also need answers to questions on whether treatment alters the natural history of the prostate cancer. Appendix 8 lists information about some of the clinical studies in progress.

Overdetection is the greatest problem of screening. This gives us the big discrepancy between latent and clinical cancer and leaves little doubt that we are identifying men who have little chance of ever getting clinical prostate cancer, or dying from it if it is untreated. Without a reliable way to predict the aggressiveness of the cancer cells, we would be treating many men who will derive no benefit at all and would suffer from the potential side effects of therapy. To further support critics of screening, the disease has a long natural history and a low death rate. The economic burden for screening, patient education, treatment of complications, primary and secondary therapy, and follow-up care also needs to be considered.

Screening is associated with benefits as well as problems. In order to reduce the death rate by 3 percent, we need to identify the cancer in 6 percent of all men. The use of the PSA annually may identify enough men to achieve this goal, but the identified cancer must be one of the aggressive types that will cause death. Most studies suggest that screening programs identify those cancers exhibiting the greatest malignant potential and support the value of prostate cancer screening.

Whether universal screening results in less death remains to be seen. But it must be remembered that nearly 60 percent of men whose cancer is detected only by a DRE have already advanced disease, whereas only about a third of those whose cancer was detected after an increase in their PSA have advanced disease. This information by itself appears to be a good reason for screening. Obviously, the clinical trials will help solve this dilemma.

Whatever is finally decided about the usefulness of PSA for prostate cancer screening, once prostate cancer has been diagnosed PSA becomes a very important yardstick for monitoring the effects of treatment on the progress of the disease. It is imperative to keep tabs on the PSA level, and you will find more about this topic in Chapter 19.

7

Grading and Staging

Two vital things to know about prostate cancer are how aggressive it is and if and how far it has spread. The pathologist's study of the cells taken from a clinical biopsy will determine how aggressive the cancer cells are. This information together with diagnostic test results help determine the variables of prostate cancer and can influence prognosis. They help guide the patient and his doctors in treatment decision making. They can arrive at a stage for the cancer. However, this stage could change later if surgery is done, and the prostate itself as well as lymph nodes are examined by the pathologist.

The Gleason Score

The pathologist is an important part of the treatment team. This is a physician who studies histology, the architecture of human tissue (glands and cells) under the microscope. The pathologist looks at the size and shape of cells and how they arrange themselves in a group.

The process of cells forming into patterns is called differentiation. Cells appearing close to normal and well organized architecturally are well differentiated and in general are slow-growing. Prostate cancer cells that are more disorganized and chaotic, forming abnormal or bizarre patterns, are poorly differentiated. These cells are usually more aggressive. It is between these two extremes that a grading system is determined. The pathologist looks for primary and secondary glandular patterns of the prostate cancer and then assigns a number from 1 to 5 to each of these two patterns. The sum of these two scores is the Gleason score. Prostate cancer cells are graded with the Gleason scoring system, named for the doctor who devised it.

For example, if the primary pattern is a 2 and the secondary pattern is a 4, then the Gleason score is six (2 + 4 = 6), indicating a moderately aggressive cancer. Scores from 8 to 10 indicate a generally more aggressive cancer. Most prostate cancer cells fall somewhere in the middle, as moderately differentiated tumors. The highest possible score is 10 (7 + 3 or 6 + 4 or 9 + 1) and the lowest is 2 (1 + 1). Remember, there are two sets of numbers, each from 1 to 5.

- **Gleason score 2 to 4.** Well-differentiated tumor; cells and glands are orderly and not chaotic.
- **Gleason score 5 to 7.** Moderately differentiated tumor, varying in size and shape; cells are beginning to invade nearby prostate tissue. This is the most common grade of prostate cancer.
- **Gleason score 8 to 10.** At this level, cells are unable to form normal patterns. They are poorly differentiated or undifferentiated, with highly irregular, distorted shapes. Cells are unable to form in regular glandular units and may have already invaded neighboring tissue. Cancer cells bear no resemblance to normal prostate cells.

In general, the lower the score, the better the response to treatment, but keep in mind that this scoring is only a guideline and is only part of the picture. Further histologic studies are done after surgery.

Results of other tests are also factored into the prognosis. If nothing showed up on CAT and bone scans, for example, it might now be determined there is no evidence of metastasis even with a moderate PSA. If a man in his 70s has a Gleason score showing a well-differentiated and slow-growing cancer, and his tumor is confined to the prostate, watchful waiting may be an acceptable option. On the other hand, if tests for a 50-year-old show that his tumor is close to the wall of the prostate, and the Gleason score is high, then his treatment choice might be surgery, so that lymph nodes and the prostate itself can be evaluated and removed for further study.

The TNM System

In addition to the Gleason score, staging for prostate cancer is usually calculated with the TNM system–tumor, nodes, metastasis. Physicians use this system when identifying the extent of disease in connection with staging. Each T category from 1 to 4 has subcategories from A to C to pinpoint the tumor more precisely. For example, a T2-A tumor occupies only one lobe of the prostate. If a 0 follows a letter, there is no evidence of cancer in that category. For example, T0 means no evidence of tumor. N0 means no evidence of cancer in the lymph nodes, and M0 means no metastasis was found.

Keep in mind that a prostate "tumor" is not removed and measured in its entirety the way it is with some other cancers. For example, when a biopsy for breast cancer is done, the nodule itself can be removed. In a prostate the tumor is not removed unless the entire prostate is removed.

- **T0.** No tumor is evident.
- **T1-A.** A tumor is not palpable on a DRE, found incidentally on TURP. Equal to less than 5 percent of the volume of tissue resected is cancerous.
- **T1-B.** Same as above, but more than 5 percent of tissue removed is cancerous.
- **T1-C.** A tumor that cannot be felt on DRE, identified by needle biopsy due to elevated PSA.
- **T2-A.** A tumor occupies less than half of one lobe of the prostate.
- **T2-B.** A tumor involves more than half of one lobe but not both lobes.
- **T2-C.** A tumor involves both lobes.
- **T3, T4.** Palpable prostate cancer that has spread outside prostate wall or into the seminal vesicles.
- **N0.** No cancer is found in the lymph nodes.
- **N+.** Cancer has spread to the lymph nodes.
- **M0.** There is no sign of distant metastases.
- **M+.** There are distant metastases to the bone.

Staging

Everything the doctors have learned about your prostate cancer–without actual surgery–from its physical appearance through all the tests is classified and subclassified: size, type, location of tumor, cell activity. All of these variables, of course, can be confusing, but because staging is not yet perfect, it is wise to be thorough. Most pathologists and urologists will rely on the staging from the Gleason scores and the TNM system. However, there are always situations that may fall between two categories, so it is sometimes a judgment call on the part of the physicians. Ask your urologist to explain how the staging was determined.

Upstaging and Downstaging

If you and your physician decide on surgical treatment, your staging may change because more prostate tissue can be studied by the pathologist. The stage of the cancer could go up or down depending on what is discovered once the prostate is removed, the lymph nodes are analyzed, and the surgeon has a chance to visually examine the area around the prostate.

For example, if a clinical biopsy shows a moderately differentiated cancer and a T2-A tumor, but after surgery it is discovered that cancer has spread to the lymph nodes, the stage will go up to N+.

The stage of prostate cancer can sometimes be lowered by hormonal treatment before surgery or radiation. Some urologists do this downstaging for 2 or 3 months to shrink the tumor and the prostate itself before surgery or radiation. Some physicians believe it is easier to operate when the cancer is smaller, but the use of hormonal downstaging is currently controversial. The chapters on surgery and radiation discuss this topic.

The Clinical Biopsy Report

The clinical biopsy report will tell you about the cells in the prostate. If prostate surgery is done, subsequent operative reports will evaluate the lymph nodes and the prostate itself. It should take no more than 7 days from the time of biopsy until receipt of the report. Doctors often hear a preliminary report from the pathologist by phone, so you may be able to learn some information sooner.

Pathology laboratories send reports to your urologist, who will explain them to you, but some doctors may not tell you everything, thinking the details are of no interest or that you would not understand them. Ask what everything means in these reports, and how your doctor interprets them. Take copies with you when you talk with other doctors for additional opinions.

Health Insurance and Biopsy

Health maintenance organizations (HMOs) often require that biopsies be done only by certain laboratories with whom they have contracts, which may not be the place your doctor has chosen to have your pathologic study done. It is also not uncommon for your surgeon to be part of your medical plan coverage, but not the laboratory he or she uses for diagnostic tests, even if the surgeon and laboratory are in the same medical center.

Let's say you have a clinical biopsy in the outpatient diagnostic center of a hospital, but your insurer will only pay for pathology done by an outside commercial laboratory, not the lab at the hospital. If you plan to receive treatment in a comprehensive cancer center, your physician will not be able to make a treatment decision based on a report from an outside commercial lab. Such laboratories are often acceptable for blood tests or analysis of potassium levels, but many doctors will not trust them for anything as critical as a tissue biopsy for cancer cells.

Current health insurance trends often fail to recognize the multidisciplinary teams that are built on mutual trust, comparable training, and professional competence. This unit can be fragmented if one or more physicians necessary for your care are not covered in your plan. Your relationship with your doctor can be strained, and access to what is perceived as necessary or desirable by health care providers is limited by health insurance coverage. Tests can cost hundreds of dollars. You and your doctor may be able to negotiate with the insurance carrier or with the pathology laboratory.

Just as the choice of pathology laboratory could be limited by your health insurance coverage, your choice of pathologist could also be limited by your physician or the hospital. Rarely are you asked to choose your own pathologist or laboratory.

When You Want a Second Pathology Opinion

Pathology laboratories have been known to make mistakes, so talk it over with your urologist if your pathology report seems out of line with other tests or if you want to double-check results. Get another opinion if your cancer has been defined as clinically insignificant—less than 0.2 centimeters—but you have a moderate Gleason score. Pathology laboratories handle hundreds of tissue samples and staff members are sometimes rushed. Ask your urologist to help you arrange for your slides to be reviewed by different pathologists to obtain a second or even third opinion on what to do next.

Tissue samples are kept on glass slides in paraffin blocks and filed away in the laboratory's pathology department. They are part of your medical record and you can have them sent to another pathologist. Hospital laboratories keep these tissue samples for many years. You will probably have to give the laboratory 24 hours' notice in writing or sign a form so they can release the slides and a written report.

PART THREE

Treatment for Early Localized Prostate Cancer

8

Watchful Waiting

Because prostate cancer is not always fatal, a man 70 or older with a slow-growing cancer who has the temperament to live with cancer in his body may be an excellent candidate for watchful waiting. This does not imply that the cancer is not treated but rather it will be treated expectantly when symptoms arise.

Naturally, there are exceptions to all rules and each man is unique. Some men in their 70s are much stronger and healthier than some men in their 50s, which must be considered. But in general the difference between the ages of 50 and 80 (assuming a cancer doubling time of 4 years) is that there are seven doubling times for the cancer cells. Watchful waiting would be a much riskier option for a younger man. The chance that the tumor will spread during his lifetime is much greater. Remember that the best opportunity to cure a man of prostate cancer is when the disease is localized to the prostate.

A 76-year-old retired diplomatic liaison who chose this option more than 4 years ago is still doing fine with no symptoms or changes in his lifestyle. When he discovered prostate cancer, he had a T2-A tumor, a Gleason score of 5 (3 + 2), and a PSA of 8. Bone and CT scans showed no metastasis. His cancer was confined to the prostate, but there was no way of knowing if it would stay there or how aggressive it might become. He had a history of hypertension treated with medications. He decided he did not want hormonal treatment or radiation. He would not have been a candidate for surgery because of his advanced age.

This man's attitude was philosophical. He was enjoying his life and did not want to risk changing that with the possible side effects of radiation or hormonal therapy. Now 80, his PSA is 14, but he has no symptoms and is still content. Bone and CT scans once again show no sign of metastasis.

This is the primary gamble of this choice. If your cancer's aggressiveness has been miscalculated, the disease might spread faster than assumed. Clinical estimates of the extent and aggressiveness of cancer cells are not 100 percent accurate. Your particular cancer could be resistant to hormone therapy aimed at slowing the cancer's growth. Another risk factor is the possibility that you may become ill from other conditions, such as heart disease or stroke, which will mean that should you choose to have surgery if your cancer grows, you may no longer be a good candidate for this treatment. The highest death rates from prostate cancer are in Scandinavia where the wait and watch approach is preferred.

Watchful waiting is not the same as doing nothing. You could decide to wait a year and use hormone therapy to slow the progress of the disease during that time. You can also change your diet as a way of possibly slowing the progress of the cancer, avoiding a high intake of animal fat and adding more fresh fruits, vegetables, and grains. This plan is not a "do nothing" choice. It means you will religiously monitor your disease through regular PSAs and DREs, and treat symptoms as they develop.

Controversy of Early Treatment

Before any man can choose to watchfully wait, he needs to understand the controversy surrounding treatment of early localized prostate cancer. He needs some idea of the chances for cure and/or recurrence of the cancer with more aggressive treatment such as surgery and radiation to compare with the more conservative choice of watchfully waiting. Are his chances better or worse?

Despite hundreds of articles and treatment regimens, the appropriate treatment for early-stage prostate cancer remains controversial. Surgical and radiation studies are hampered by an inadequate staging system. We don't have enough clinical trials and long-term studies. The disease itself adds to the dilemma with its long natural history and slow doubling time.

Surgical studies have often reported results based on pathological staging done after surgery. Radiation studies have not had the advantage of removing patients with positive nodes or extracapsular disease from the studies. Patients have different PSA levels. These factors make direct comparison of surgery with radiation difficult.

Gleason grade and stage have been historically reported as the most important pretreatment factors for predicting the outcome for early-stage cancer. However, directly comparing surgical and radiation outcomes on the basis of stage alone is fraught with problems because patients with higher PSA and grade are more frequently treated with radiation therapy, either external or internal. Several recent surgical and radiation studies have indicated that PSA levels before treatment may be more significant than either grade or stage as an objective prognostic factor. Grade also appears to be an important factor.

How do you measure a successful treatment outcome? Normalization of the PSA? The fact that the patient is still alive? But couldn't the patient have been incompletely treated and still be alive? In recent years, it has been more difficult to analyze outcomes of prostate cancer treatment. In the past, local control was established by performing a periodic DRE to look for evidence of recurrence. However, it can take a decade or more for cancer to become detectable this way, so we look to more sensitive parameters through biopsy after treatment or by following the PSA levels. The rise in PSA following treatment is considered biochemical evidence of either local failure or progression of the disease.

Degrees of Difference in Early Cancer

Cancer that has been staged at T1 with the TNM (tumor, nodes, metastasis) system (see Chapter 7) is early and localized within the prostate. But it is important to distinguish between the degrees of this stage: A, B, and C. Men with T1-A have low-volume and low-grade tumors, with little likelihood of the disease progressing any time soon. The cancer is equal to or less than 5 percent of the volume of the prostate tissue removed after transurethral resection of the prostate (TURP) and the Gleason score is between 2 and 5.

In contrast, T1-B means there is a slightly higher volume and grade of cancer present. This stage is comparable to T2-A. The cancer is more than 5 percent of the volume of the prostate and the Gleason score may be between 6 and 10. Men with either of these stages have a higher risk that the disease will progress and metastasize.

Men with cancers staged at T1-A might probably be safe with watchful waiting. Patients with T1-B tumors are like T2-A and more aggressive therapy may be warranted. The number of men diagnosed with T1-C disease has increased markedly since the introduction of PSA screening. There are many latent cancers in this group and clinical outcome should be based on tumor grade, volume, and diagnostic tests.

Although there are obvious benefits of detecting more organ-confined prostate cancer, there is still major controversy about the large numbers of men with clinically insignificant cancer staged at T1-C. Johns Hopkins University researchers examined the pathological results of men who had radical prostatectomies and who had been staged as T1-C before treatment. After study of the prostate specimens, the staging remained about the same. Most were between stage T1-A and T2. The tumors were confined to the prostate, their Gleason scores were less than 7, and the tumors were small.

Such minimal tumors were found in 16 percent of stage T1-C patients. The cancer was confined to the prostate in half of the men. Almost 20 percent had cancer that had progressed to the wall of the prostate. Therefore, stage T1-C represents a different kind of tumor. Thus, whereas 20 percent may have had cancer that would not progress, some men had evidence of a significant but potentially curable cancer with surgery. Obviously, we need a reliable means of distinguishing between low-volume indolent tumors and those that will progress. The importance of using PSA density and velocity, as well as Gleason score and cancer volume, is obvious.

Studies thus far reporting results of watchful waiting or conservative management are flawed by design, but it is clear that most men with well-differentiated cancer will not die from the cancer 10 years later. This finding suggests overall survival in men with a life expectancy of 10 years or less and who have many other health problems; these men are unlikely to benefit from aggressive treatment of early prostate cancer.

However, the risk of progression to metastatic cancer in 10 years is approximately 40 percent in men being treated with watchful waiting with moderately differentiated tumors. Although these men avoid the side effects of radiation and radical prostatectomy, many are likely to suffer from side effects from secondary symptoms such as urinary problems if the disease progresses. In addition to hormonal therapy, which can be palliative for bone pain, some may also need surgery to relieve bladder obstruction.

Men who are diagnosed with early localized cancer face difficult choices. Conflicting studies and reports that are often incomplete or biased in the media add to the confusion. It is important to be fully informed about the pros and cons of surgery and radiation before considering the option of watchful waiting.

9

Surgery: Radical Prostatectomy

Radical prostatectomy is performed when prostate cancer has not spread beyond the prostate. Don't let the word *radical* scare you. It describes the removal of the entire prostate, seminal vesicles, and lymph nodes that drain the prostate. With some cancers, only part of the diseased organ is removed. For instance, with colon cancer, only the diseased section of the colon needs to be removed, and there are mastectomies that do not remove the entire breast. The transurethral resection known as the TURP is also a form of prostatectomy, but it is used only to remove tissue of the transition zone or inner core of the prostate when benign prostatic hyperplasia (BPH) is present. Once there is known cancer, the entire gland must be removed.

In the past, prostatectomies left all men impotent and most men incontinent because the muscles, nerves, and blood vessels vital to these functions are so close to the prostate. The relationship of these structures to each other was not fully appreciated, so they were very commonly injured during surgery. Surgical techniques have improved considerably, but there is still a risk for both incontinence and impotence after radical prostatectomy, although permanent urinary incontinence is now extremely rare and impotence can be overcome with medical alternatives.

In 1988, surgeons at Johns Hopkins University developed the anatomic technique for radical prostate surgery so that the neurovascular sheaths, also called bundles, alongside the prostate are not injured during surgery. This nerve-sparing radical prostatectomy is now widely used but is still controversial, because some surgeons believe that when they avoid these bundles, they risk leaving cancer behind and there is the theoretical potential of a higher risk of recurrence.

Surgical treatment has increased dramatically in recent years, as we are finding cancer in younger men because of early detection with PSA. More patients under 70 are now identified with stage T1-C disease. Before 1994, with only the DRE as a diagnostic tool, the cancer was usually inoperable by the time it was found.

Surgery is usually recommended as a curative treatment for all early prostate cancer, when the tumor is confined to the prostate, the PSA is less than 10, and the patient is under 70 years of age (or has a greater than 10-year life expectancy) and has no other medical conditions, such as heart or lung disease, that put him at risk for higher postoperative complications. After prostatectomy, PSA should decrease to almost undetectable levels because without the prostate it is no longer being produced.

Technique of Radical Prostatectomy

Prostate surgery can be performed through an incision in the lower abdomen or through the perineum, the area between the scrotum and the anus. The perineal approach was first practiced in 1858 and the abdominal approach was developed in 1947. The abdominal approach allows more room to work so that the urologist can remove the prostate and examine the pelvic area, including the lymph nodes. The key to success in prostate surgery is being able to see everything clearly.

When the prostate is surgically removed, a small amount of tissue around the prostate is also removed in order to determine if any cancer has grown beyond the prostate. This border is called a margin, and you will hear about it as a positive margin or a negative margin. If any part of the margin is positive, it means cancer has reached that border and possibly has already gone farther. And if the margin is negative, it means there is a cancer-free border around the prostate. The chance that cancer cells have traveled elsewhere is lessened. The margins exist at the level of the bladder neck and urethra, two places where the prostate is cut away from the body. To achieve negative margins, the urologist may have to remove some of the delicate muscles that help control urinary function and some of the nerves that assist in producing erections. Some doctors want wide margins around the prostate to be safe. The nerve-sparing surgery requires leaving a narrower margin around the prostate to avoid injuring the nerves.

The sheath containing the neurovascular bundles is on both sides of the prostate. More than half of prostate cancer escapes from the gland in this area. The decision of whether to take out the neurovascular bundles to develop a wide excision is made at the time of surgery. If the disease is palpable on the ipsilateral side, the same side where the tumor was noted on biopsy, then most urologists would recommend taking the neurovascular bundle out.

With an abdominal incision, the surgeon has the opportunity to sample the lymph nodes so that the pathologist can examine with a microscope whether the cancer has spread. Lymph nodes are generally removed and checked for the presence of cancer before the prostate is removed. If the lymph nodes are positive, then the prostate is not removed because there is no opportunity to locally control the disease with surgery.

The Retropubic Approach

Most prostate surgery in the United States is done with the retropubic technique—an incision in the lower abdomen between the navel and the pubic bone.

Retro means "behind," and by making an incision in the lower abdomen, the urologist can reach into the pelvic area from behind the pubic bone. From this entry, the urologist can gently move aside the intestines, bladder, and other organs, and visually examine the entire area for anything suspicious. The urologist can remove lymph nodes and leave wide margins as the prostate is surgically removed.

After dividing the urethra, the surgeon separates the prostate from the rectum, then divides the bladder neck. The prostate specimen with the seminal vesicles is then removed with care and the connections from the kidney to the bladder, called ureters, are inspected to make sure they are not injured during the dissection. The bladder neck and urethra are then joined with sutures. This connection is called an anastomosis.

The Nerve-Sparing Technique

This technique also uses the same retropubic approach through an incision in the lower abdomen. The outcome of any surgery—but especially this one—depends on the skill of the surgeon and his or her knowledge of anatomy.

The goal is to preserve the nerves responsible for erections. These are in two sheaths called neurovascular bundles leaning right up against either side of the prostate. Sometimes, even if only one of these bundles can be saved, impotence is avoided, especially in younger men. If the operation spares one bundle, it is called unilateral. It is bilateral if both are spared.

Some urologists are unwilling to leave behind any tissue that may be harboring cancer cells, and they assume that if the cancer has progressed to one neurovascular bundle, it is probably in the other one as well. They will remove both sides. The area of the prostate where the bundles lie cannot be felt during a DRE, so when the urologist exposes the prostate during surgery and the prostate feels hard with tumor close to the nerves, the nerve-sparing procedure generally will not be done.

There is much controversy here, even about the accuracy of some of the studies. It is critical that you ask your urologist to be frank about how many of these nerve-sparing surgeries he or she has performed, what complications have been encountered, as well as how many patients retained their potency.

Attempting to prevent impotence with this technique also increases the chances of cutting into cancer cells. Half of all cancers that escape from the prostate go into the spaces that surround these nerves. Examination of hundreds of radical prostatectomy specimens in clinical studies found that the nerve-sparing operation exposes men to a serious risk of leaving cancer cells behind. Reports on the incidence of positive surgical margins vary, but as more and more urologists employ this technique and carefully select patients for the procedure, the positive surgical margin rate is decreasing.

The Perineal Approach

The prostate gland can also be removed through an incision made in the perineum, the region between the scrotum and the anus. With this approach, a patient spends less time under anesthesia, and therefore the operating time is shorter. For an obese man with a small prostate gland, it may also be a better surgical approach.

The prostate is approached from a different angle, however, and only a relatively small prostate can be removed this way because the opening is comparatively small. If your prostate is very enlarged, it might not be easily done. The perineal technique does not allow for the removal of lymph nodes, which may need to be removed either ahead of time laparoscopically through the abdomen or later through traditional surgery. If that is the case, the hospital time is extended to more than a week. Another drawback is that the surgeon cannot see if any other cancer is apparent. This "gross" examination is often an important part of surgery.

This technique is a better one for bladder neck reconstruction. There is usually less blood loss and a shorter recovery time—usually 2 days in the hospital.

Shrinking the Tumor Before Surgery

Some physicians may recommend 2 or 3 months of hormonal treatment (neoadjuvant therapy) before surgery to shrink the tumor or the prostate itself. The production of testosterone can be reduced with an androgen blockade and the prostate can be examined with ultrasound to document the reduced size. By reducing the volume of the tumor—or downstaging the cancer—some physicians believe they also reduce some of the risks of surgery such as blood loss and length of time on the operating table. They feel the chance for positive surgical margins is also reduced.

A random study of 100 patients, some of whom were given leuprolide (Lupron) before surgery to block testosterone production, showed a 50 percent reduction in positive margins after radical prostatectomy for those who took Lupron. This study suggested that the androgen deprivation before surgery caused a downstaging of the tumor, for example, from stage T3 to T2. Biologically, how downstaging occurs with androgen deprivation is still unknown.

Dr. Ferdinand LaBrie, of the CHUL Research Center at L'Hotel Dieu de Quebec, studied a group of men having surgery alone and another group taking Lupron and flutamide (Eulexin) before surgery. His studies showed the positive margin rate was significantly lower with the neoadjuvant treatment group.

Other physicians believe shrinking the tumor makes the surgery more difficult because it distorts the normal anatomical planes. They also argue that you cannot make a tumor go back into the prostate once it has already spread outside. If it has grown large, the cancer cells are already multiplying elsewhere, so it is argued that neoadjuvant hormonal manipulation prior to surgery makes no biological sense.

Neoadjuvant treatment is still investigational in 1997 because there are no long-term studies to indicate longer survival time. We have no proof yet that even though the tumor has been reduced and the margins are negative after surgery, a cancer cell or cells have not already traveled to other organs to take residence and grow.

Risks of Prostatectomy

Any major surgery carries complication risks. Blood clots can form in the veins during or after surgery, causing a deep venous thrombosis or pulmonary embolus (clot traveling to the lung). The incidence of this problem is low—less than 3 percent—but the risk increases with age and is naturally higher if you have a history of cardiopulmonary problems. You are at higher risk for surgery if you smoke, drink, or have a chronic illness such as heart, lung, gastrointestinal problems, or diabetes. If you are overweight or emotionally stressed, your risk for complications is higher.

Your health has an impact on follow-up treatment, too. Ask your prostate cancer treatment team members to consult with your family doctor or other medical specialists who treat you.

To prevent the need for a blood transfusion from an unknown donor, you may donate your own blood before surgery. This procedure is known as an autologous blood donation.

Rectal injury sometimes occurs because the back of the rectum is close to the prostate, but this injury is found in less than 1 percent of patients. When it does occur, a primary repair can be performed or a colostomy is temporarily constructed to divert the colon and fecal stream to a bag outside the body until the rectum heals.

The urethral channel in the area of the anastomosis becomes too narrow in 5 to 10 percent of cases. This urethral stricture impedes the flow of urine and it can usually be relieved with a dilation procedure performed in your physician's office.

The most feared risks of prostate surgery are incontinence and impotence. (There are chapters devoted to overcoming these conditions in Part VI of this book.) Studies from the Prostate Disease Patient Outcomes

Research Team of the U.S. Agency for Health Care Policy and Research found about 25 percent of men experienced some form of urinary incontinence after surgery, and 85 percent noticed changes in sexual function.

Incontinence

Everyone is incontinent for a while after a radical prostatectomy. Incontinence can last for a few days or a few months, but with special exercises, behavior modification, and sometimes with medications, normal continence is eventually restored in most men.

The internal sphincter muscle that automatically controls the flow of urine is damaged when the prostate is removed and the urethra is sewn directly to the bladder neck. The internal sphincter muscles are part of a ring of muscles around the bladder neck. Once the internal sphincter is gone, all the work of starting and stopping the flow of urine must be done by the external sphincter located on the pelvic floor. Until this muscle is strengthened again, about 35 percent of patients experience a degree of stress incontinence, which happens when you cough or sneeze or change position from sitting to standing. Other types of incontinence include urge incontinence, which means you feel the urge to urinate that is so extreme you might leak if you do not urinate right away. Overflow incontinence is caused by an obstruction such as BPH where you are "flowing over the top." Global incontinence means you have absolutely no control, that you are leaking urine all the time. This condition is extremely rare after prostatectomy, occurring in less than 3 percent of patients 12 months after radical prostatectomy.

Impotence

Impotence occurs because nerves and blood vessels necessary for erection are injured or severed during surgery. Impotence means you cannot achieve or maintain a rigid erection. It does not mean you cannot achieve orgasm or that you lose the desire for sex. Based on various studies, your age and potency before the operation have a great deal to do with your outcome after radical prostatectomy.

If you are over 70, it may be unrealistic to think you will be potent following radical prostatectomy. But most men can figure on the following averages, assuming nerves were spared on both sides of the prostate:

- If you are in your 70s, you have a 30 percent chance of return of potency.
- If you are in your 60s, you have a 50 percent chance.
- If you are in your 50s, you have a 70 percent chance.
- If you are in your 40s, you have more than an 80 percent chance.

Refer to Chapter 18 for ways to restore potency.

Lymphadenectomy: Removing Lymph Nodes

Lymph nodes are small glands that act as filters in the body's drainage system and they are encased in fatty tissue in strategic locations throughout your body. Lymphatic fluid flows upward from the prostate. Some nodes are like heavy bunches of grapes. Others are spread out and far apart like marbles dropped on the floor. Some nodes are like tiny seeds; others are more like jelly beans. Sometimes lymph nodes are enlarged, either from infection or inflammation, or if they are filled with cancer cells.

It is possible for lymph nodes to be cancer-free even in the presence of a fairly large prostate carcinoma, but it is much less likely. It is also possible for lymph nodes to be enlarged and show no cancer. If the cancer has spread to the lymph nodes, it means there is a greater chance it has escaped into other parts of the body.

Traditional Technique

When the prostate is removed, the urologist will also dissect the lymph nodes—usually three or six from either side of the prostate. Lymphadenectomy is critical not only for staging; it is also believed by some to be therapeutic. If any lymph nodes contain cancer, then their removal has eliminated additional cancer from the body.

Once the fatty tissue containing the lymph nodes is surgically removed, the pathologist examines the tissue. Normally, a pathologist is standing by to quickly analyze a frozen section of the nodes under the microscope. This analysis takes a few minutes and is done in the lab or in the operating room. Each dissected lymph node is examined carefully by the pathologist for the final pathology report.

If the frozen section shows cancer, most urologists will not proceed with the radical prostatectomy, since now that the horse is already out of the barn, removing the prostate will not provide a cure. They will close up the incision and suggest treatment with hormones. However, even if the lymph nodes are negative–showing no cancer–a small number of men can still develop evidence of metastatic disease over time because the cancer had begun to escape the prostate gland prior to surgery but was too microscopic to be detected by preoperative staging.

Laparoscopic Technique

A laparoscopic lymphadenectomy can be performed in the hospital before the prostatectomy. This procedure is expensive and most doctors use it only when they are already pretty sure the cancer has spread and they want to confirm that diagnosis in order to spare the patient further surgery. This type of investigation of the lymph nodes is generally done in men with a T3 or T4 tumor who are contemplating surgery or external beam radiation treatment.

Several small incisions are made in the abdomen and a scope with a video camera attached is inserted into the pelvic area. By watching a monitor, the urologist can guide the scope to the lymph nodes and with special tools the lymph nodes are removed and sent to the pathologist for analysis. If there is no cancer in the lymph nodes after laparoscopic dissection, some urologists will go ahead with the radical prostatectomy immediately, but some will schedule the surgery for another day.

Laparoscopic lymphadenectomy is not commonly used because it requires two procedures. It is much more efficient to do traditional surgery and remove the lymph nodes at the same time.

Pathology of the Prostate Specimen

Once the prostate gland is removed from your body, it is no longer called a prostate but is now called a prostate specimen. For the surgical specimen after radical prostatectomy, pathologists examine separately the prostate, lymph nodes, and seminal vesicles, looking for cancer cells. This examination serves as the basis for the final staging of the disease, the so-called pathological stage. If the stage changes from the earlier clinical biopsy, it more commonly goes up rather than down.

The pathologist plays a critical role in your surgery. A careful and deliberate pathologist will analyze the prostate and lymph nodes with great care. When the prostate is removed, the pathologist puts ink around the gland. There are actually two cut ends: one at the apex, where the prostate joins the urethra, and one at the base, the bladder neck.

The prostate is sliced into sections that are meticulously examined under the microscope. Evaluation is made whether or not the cancer cells are near the edges of the slices or appear to have already penetrated those edges or margins. When the pathologist slices into the prostate specimen, he or she can check each slice to see if any cancer cells have reached the inked margin.

When cancer is confined to the prostate and has not reached the margins, fewer than one patient in 10 has a recurrence. Recurrence is more likely if cancer has spread to the margins. In this case, with cure unlikely, palliative treatment with hormones or radiation is considered.

If the cancer has penetrated the fat around the prostate, there is generally a 60 percent chance of recurrence in 5 years. If it has penetrated the seminal vesicles, the chance increases to 86 percent, and if it has gone into the lymph nodes, the chance is 97 percent.

The Pathology Report

The pathologist's report will usually be available within five business days, so you may be out of the hospital before the results are known. This report will have a great bearing on your prognosis and whether future treatment is needed. It is the pathological staging.

Pathologists have a certain agenda to follow when investigating prostate cancer, according to the Association of Directors of Anatomic and Surgical Pathology. Your pathology report should include:

- A description of the tumor in terms of percentage of tumor in relation to the amount of prostate tissue that is not cancerous
- The presence of tumor at the surgical margins
- The site of an extracapsular tumor involvement

- The presence or absence of carcinoma in the neurovascular bundles
- The presence or absence of carcinoma in the seminal vesicles
- Metastasis in the lymph nodes

This analysis is one of your most important medical reports and it is a good idea to become familiar with it while you are undergoing treatment. Be sure to ask for a copy so that you can show it to your other physicians.

When Margins Are Positive

About 40 to 50 percent of men who have a radical prostatectomy for T1 or T2 disease have positive surgical margins, which means residual cancer cells may be lurking in the area. The most common sites are the apex and the base near the bladder neck. It is highly likely that if the margins are positive, the cancer has penetrated the capsule of the prostate. However, it may take many years for the cancer to recur or become detectable, so the PSA must be monitored faithfully.

The PSA of a 52-year-old man who had positive margins after a radical prostatectomy began to rise 4 years after surgery. A CAT (computerized axial tomography) scan showed a tiny nodule in the area where the prostate had been and biopsy confirmed that it was cancer. This patient opted for external beam radiation treatment and his PSA has since decreased to very low levels.

Treatment of men with positive margins is also controversial. Positive margins may indicate a need for adjuvant therapy after surgery. Also to be considered are the patient's age and medical condition and the possibilities of complications from further treatment. Treatment options include radiation or hormonal treatment as well as watchful surveillance including serial DRE and PSA tests.

Another question is whether to begin treatment right after surgery or to wait until symptoms appear. A detailed workup should be done including PSA levels and possibly bone and CAT scans, or an ultrasound-guided biopsy. If the PSA is rising but the other tests are negative, with no indication of a site of recurrence, then the options are to either follow the PSA and treat the patient with hormones when they become symptomatic or start early hormonal therapy prior to the onset of symptoms.

If the PSA is rising and the biopsy is positive showing local recurrence but there is no metastasis, then radiation or hormonal therapy could be offered. If the PSA is rising and there is evidence of metastasis on bone or CAT scans, hormonal therapy is the wisest choice.

The Risk of Recurrence

We have no long-term studies with meaningful data on prostate cancer recurrence rates after surgical treatment. Does surgery add years to your life? The jury is still out. Because prostate cancer grows so slowly, researchers need to follow patients for at least 15 years to determine if a treatment is effective. A 1992 study found that when cancer did not escape the confines of the prostate, only 2 percent of men had local recurrences within 5 years after radical retropubic prostatectomy and 1 percent had distant metastases. A Medicare survey of older men showed 28 percent had recurrence after radical prostatectomy. Overall, the recurrence rate is about 12 percent.

Recurrence means the cancer reappears in the same region—where the prostate used to be. In contrast, metastatic prostate cancer means the cancer appears outside the prostate area, such as in the bone, liver, or lung. The treatment of recurrent prostate cancer is highly individual. Palliative treatment with radiation or hormonal therapy is an option.

Some investigators suggest that if you are 65 or younger, you will live an average of 14 months longer by choosing surgery instead of watchful waiting. The National Cancer Institute has initiated a long-term study—the Prostate Cancer Intervention Versus Observation Trial (PIVOT)—to find out if surgery is really more effective than doing nothing.

Questions to Ask About Surgery

• **Please describe the operation.**
It is important that your urologist describe the way the surgery will be performed so that you understand the technique used and whether the plan is to spare the nerves needed for potency.

• **Will any nerves or blood vessels be damaged?**

Even with the nerve-sparing technique, it is possible that some may be damaged. For example, if the cancer is close to one of the neurovascular bundles, those may be severed, leaving you with only one bundle intact. Obviously, you need to understand this possibility before surgery.

• **If nerves are spared, is the risk of recurrence of prostate cancer greater?**

Some studies have indicated that there is a greater chance of recurrence of prostate cancer in men who have had the nerve-sparing surgery. In the meantime, urologists are gaining more experience and skill and this surgical technique has improved since its early days.

• **What are the side effects of surgery?**

Naturally, the two major side effects are the possibilities of urinary incontinence and/or impotence. Each man is unique and your doctor should tell you how much of those side effects to expect. However, there may be other side effects to consider, too, such as psychological issues, depression, and quality of life.

• **Will you remove any lymph nodes?**

It is generally standard procedure to remove some of the lymph nodes around the prostate if a radical prostatectomy is performed. This provides more information about whether or not the cancer has begun to spread outside the prostate.

• **If you find cancer in the lymph nodes, will treatment change?**

Yes, it is possible your prostate will not be removed if the lymph nodes are shown to contain cancer. During the operation a frozen section of the nodes may be done, which means the pathologist does an on-the-spot examination of the nodes to find out if cancer is present. A more thorough and detailed examination is done later, called a permanent section, and is part of the official pathology report.

• **How much pain will I have after surgery?**

Some men experience very little pain and others have a great deal, so find out what kinds of treatment will be available for your pain management and see the next chapter for more details about pain control during and after radical prostatectomy.

• **What kind of follow-up care will you provide?**

Most urologists will see you several times after surgery to check up on your recovery to the surgery itself. Depending on your particular case, you will always need periodic examinations and consultations with your urologist.

• **What are my options if the cancer recurs?**

Your doctor should explain the possibility of radiation or hormonal therapy if the cancer recurs.

10

Before and After Surgery

There are many procedures and layers of administrative detail to get through before surgery. The administration of health care is more complex not only because there are more patients to handle, but because the health care system itself is going through such enormous change that medical centers and physicians must keep track of every detail of a patient's care.

Hospitals process patients through surgery using a multidisciplinary approach to care that the physicians, nurses, and technicians will follow before, during, and after surgery. This approach involves interviews with you and your family, preoperative tests, medications, diet monitoring, treatments, teaching you follow-up care, and planning for discharge. While some hospitals may give you an informal photocopied sheet or two with pre-op instructions, some may give you a 15-page workbook that contains not only information and instructions about each step along the way but space for you to record your doctor's names and phone numbers, as well as procedure code numbers for your medical insurance company. (New York Hospital–Cornell Medical Center provides this type of workbook.)

The Weeks Before Surgery

There are many preparations to make before surgery, such as donating your own blood, arranging for home care, altering your use of medications, and handling health insurance concerns. If you are anticipating the need for surgery, you may want to meet with the hospital social worker or the home care staff.

Generally, a nurse will review your medical history with you and ask what medications you take. Your height, weight, and blood pressure will be recorded. This is the time to let the hospital know if you have any food or drug allergies and if you have special dietary requirements for religious or medical reasons. This preoperative process generates a great deal of paperwork, and it should all be attached to your chart when you show up for surgery. It might be a good idea to get copies yourself and bring them with you. If there is any change in your health during this preoperative period, even a cold or fever, let your doctor know about it.

Because you may be facing a few weeks or months of urinary incontinence after surgery, training in special Kegel exercises may begin during this time. See Chapter 17 for more information about these exercises.

Meeting Your Treatment Team

Before surgery, you need reassurance from your doctor. Find out if your urologist will see you before you go into the operating room. Ask what will happen in there, how many people will be working on you, how long the surgery will take, and where you will go when it is over.

Find out in advance which family member or friend will be able to talk with your surgeon once the surgery is completed. This person needs to know how you are and can relay news to other family members, and possibly your other doctors. Should that person meet your urologist in the waiting room, your hospital room, or in the doctor's office at the hospital?

Will your urologist explain what he or she has found while examining the inside of your pelvic area? Some urologists may hesitate to say they saw cancerous lymph nodes until they have the pathologist's report of the lymph node dissection, but they should tell you they are checking on any lesions they may have discovered. This is important for peace of mind for your family and will avoid frustration later when you wake up in your room and have no information.

In addition to your own urologist, there may be other attending doctors from the hospital's urology staff. Possibly a resident may visit you during daily rounds, and if you are in a teaching hospital, students and other doctors may visit.

Alerting Your Other Doctors

Let your family doctor—or doctors other than your urologist—know when surgery is planned. They may want to visit you in the hospital after surgery to see how you are doing from their perspective. If you have other ongoing medical problems, such as heart or lung conditions, it is a good idea to be followed before, during, and after your surgery by your primary care doctor, internist, or other specialist treating these conditions. These doctors may want to monitor your blood pressure, heart, kidney function, and respiratory tract to watch out for pneumonia and reactions to the medications they have prescribed for you as well as reactions to medications given during and after your surgery. These doctors should enjoy a good working relationship with your urologist.

If you have any prostheses such as a hip replacement or heart valve, you may need antibiotic prophylaxis against infection. The urologist will probably want to consult with the doctors who manage these conditions.

The Hospital Support Staff

Some hospitals routinely assign special cancer care nurses to surgery patients. Ask your doctor in advance what to expect. Will the floor nurse come whenever you need him or her or should you hire a private nurse for the first day or two? This question is particularly important if other health conditions make you more vulnerable. Before you are admitted, go to the nurses' station on the floor where you will be staying and ask the nurses how they feel about this issue, or ask a friend or family member to talk to the nurse.

The amount of time that floor nurses can give you depends on the size of the hospital, the number of nurses available in your unit, and how highly skilled they are in dealing with equipment and procedures required in your postop care. Usually there is a nurse manager for each unit, registered nurses, and patient care assistants such as nurses' aides. If the hospital medical staff members feel extra care is needed, they can give you a roster of private-duty nurses available, both registered nurses and licensed practical nurses. Consider whether you will want three nurses, each working an 8-hour shift right after your surgery, or if you would like one for the same time each day, say from 8 A.M. to 4 P.M. to help you get up and walk around, administer medications, and change dressings. Some hospital personnel are described as follows:

- Your hospital may have a blood team, which means someone will take blood samples from you each day.

- There may be an IV (intravenous) team to check on the IV lines. They are usually registered nurses.
- Social workers are part of most hospital support staffs. A social worker may help explain your insurance coverage, support groups or other emotional help, and care options after you go home.
- Patient service representatives can help you and your family with care while you are in the hospital.

Home Health Care

For the first week or so after discharge from the hospital, you may want to engage a home health worker, especially if you live alone, have complications from surgery, or have additional medical problems. Sometimes this care is helpful for older men, or for those who have an ill spouse or partner who is not able to help them. Your hospital social work department or the home health care department can arrange this care for you.

A home care nurse can check your vital signs and change your dressings each day for a week, then perhaps visit less often. With this kind of professional help, you can also relieve some anxiety and reinforce your training about your new condition, such as adapting to a urethral catheter, which is typically left in place up to 3 weeks after surgery to drain urine from your bladder.

While you are in the hospital, ask if you are eligible for this care. This area is very gray in terms of medical insurance coverage. If your doctor says you require wound care or you need help with taking your medications, or with the urethral catheter, then your medical insurance may cover the cost. There may be limitations, however, such as the number of covered visits by a nurse or home health aide. Medical insurance often covers such services because it decreases time spent in the hospital, which is much more expensive.

Before You Consent to Surgery

You may be asked to sign consent forms for surgery, biopsy, and many procedures you encounter along the way. Don't sign anything until you know exactly what will happen to you. Informed consent means you give permission when you have complete knowledge of the treatment protocol.

Generally, radical prostatectomy means your prostate, lymph nodes, and seminal vesicles will be removed and nothing else. Should you want elective surgery while you are there, such as the repair of a hernia, then that should be arranged in advance.

The entire procedure should be explained to you by your physician and health care team. You (and your family) should be educated about what to expect after surgery. Your physician can relieve some of your fears by explaining the procedures and helping you understand what you can expect from each one of them.

Advance Directive

If for any reason you should become unable to make decisions about your care, you need a way to let your physician and the hospital know what you choose to do about treatment. The advance directive, a written or oral statement, allows you to plan in advance for any eventuality that could leave you unable to communicate with your treatment team. It is your right to accept or refuse medical treatment, which includes life support systems. You have a right to request or consent to treatment, refuse treatment before it has started, or have it stopped once it has begun.

You can also appoint a proxy, a friend, or someone from your family to carry out your wishes. If you do not have an advance directive, your family may not be allowed to make decisions for you. You can outline your wishes about your treatment—and your life—in a living will. Whomever you appoint as an agent or proxy for you has the right to carry out your wishes.

Most hospitals now have a policy regarding advance directives, which are mandated by law in many states. Adult patients are usually informed of their right to make such directives when they enter the hospital.

Decisions of this magnitude should always be in writing. Most hospitals have the appropriate forms for you to complete if you have not already done so. Give a copy of your advance directive, living will, or health care proxy to your doctor and one to the hospital to keep with your medical chart.

Health Insurance Considerations

Financial data are usually confirmed prior to surgery, and you may need to talk with your insurance company about procedures ahead of time.

Health insurance companies normally require advance notification of surgery, so once your surgery has been scheduled, call and give them the date and type of surgery. They should give you an authorization number or they may call your physician for more information.

Some insurance companies do not cover all the preoperative procedures and tests because they do not consider them vital. It is critically important that you be well informed about your medical insurance and what it covers so that you can go through the procedures without worrying about coverage. Also, if you are not covered for certain procedures that are part of managing your case in the hospital, you may run into problems with the hospital.

A radical prostatectomy with lymph node dissection and follow-up care can cost thousands of dollars. Hospital and physician costs are separate. The anesthesiologist will bill you separately, but this fee may not always be covered by insurance plans. You may have to pay for blood donations you make, too.

Find out what is covered by your health plan and also find out how many months of follow-up care will be covered. Medicare and Medicaid pay for follow-up care for a certain number of months, depending on the procedures you have.

If you are confused by your insurance, always ask to talk with the hospital's social worker or patient services representative, whose job it is to help with these kinds of problems. If you have a deductible to pay on your plan before coverage begins, some hospitals may require you to pay this amount up front.

Reviewing Medications

Seven days before surgery, you will probably be asked to stop taking aspirin products such as Anacin and Bufferin, as well as anti-inflammatory agents such as Motrin, Nuprin, and Advil. Aspirin can cause increased bleeding during surgery. Tylenol is generally safe to take for headaches or other pain during this preoperative period.

At this time antibiotics may be prescribed to prepare you for surgery, because there is the slight chance the rectum can be injured and release bacteria into the surgical area. If your bowel is clean and you take an antibiotic, the risk of infection is reduced.

If you are on routine medications for a health condition, such as blood pressure or heart medications, ask your doctor if you should continue to take them before and after surgery. If you are a diabetic, your physicians will help you manage your insulin or oral medications during the hours of fasting before surgery. Iron supplements may be prescribed by your physician if you are planning to donate your own blood.

Banking Your Own Blood

Radical prostatectomy is a much less bloody operation than it used to be. However, some men may need a blood transfusion during the procedure, and it is always safer to receive a transfusion of your own blood. This autologous blood donation is collected from you three times, usually one unit of blood each week, during the month before surgery. Because blood is perishable after 45 days, you need a firm surgery date before you donate blood.

Your family or friends can also donate blood for you, which is known as a directed donation. Some patients choose both their own and directed donations. You may be able to donate only one or two units, and someone else can donate another one or two. It is always possible you will need additional blood, so ask the hospital how blood is screened for HIV (human immunodeficiency virus) and hepatitis.

If iron supplements are prescribed, you begin taking them a week before you begin donating your own blood. The iron can turn your stool black or make you constipated. A stool softener, such as Colace, can be added to your list of preoperative medications. Colace, as well as iron supplements, are available without prescription at most drugstores.

You will not be able to donate blood within 3 days of dental work because of the possibility of infection. Also, you will not be able to donate blood if you are taking antibiotics. Refrain from any strenuous activity on the day of your donation. Never give blood on an empty stomach, and drink plenty of fluids before and after giving blood.

Believe it or not, you may have to pay to donate your own blood, and you may have to pay for it up front. This "processing" charge can be as much as $100 or more, so check with your insurance carrier. Directed donations will also be subject to this charge, but it should be covered by your insurance.

Preoperative Tests

Within 2 weeks of surgery, you may be scheduled for preoperative tests such as an electrocardiogram (EKG), blood and urine tests, and a chest X-ray to check your general health and be sure you are able to tolerate surgery and anesthesia. Tests are individualized for each patient. Depending on your condition, you may need additional tests.

- An **EKG** is a normal part of the routine before surgery to check your heart function and to detect any abnormalities that may cause complications during anesthesia and surgery.
- A **chest X-ray** may be required before surgery to verify you have no pulmonary infection or signs of metastasis in your lungs.
- A **complete blood count (CBC)** to check for iron deficiency anemia is important so that this problem can be corrected before surgery.

Things to Do Before Surgery: A Checklist

Prostate cancer treatment affects your work, family, and lifestyle. If you have open abdominal surgery, for example, you may be in the hospital for 3 to 5 days, and it will take several more weeks before you are recovered enough to go back to work or to resume your daily activities. Rearrange your work and social schedule, and get ready for the surgery and your recuperation. The more you know and plan in advance, the less stress and discomfort you will experience later when you feel helpless and not in the mood to think about the details of your life.

You may want to find out ahead of time what you will need at the hospital. Will you be able to wear your own clothes? Can you get a newspaper each day? Should you bring some books or your portable CD player? What about other medications and toiletries?

- Designate someone to talk with the surgeon immediately after your surgery and to contact your other physicians about the results, such as whether lymph nodes are negative or positive.
- Ask about the equipment you need to help cope postoperatively,

such as the urethral catheter. Are you sure you know how to use it? Do you know what to do if it malfunctions?

- Find out what support systems are available to you if you find you need help coping with your feelings. There is often a feeling of letdown right after surgery.

- Arrange your work schedule so that you will know how much time off you can count on, and when and how you are likely to return to work. Arrange for someone to handle details of your work that may be necessary.

- Plan for someone to care for things at home while you are in the hospital.

The Day and Night Before Surgery

Prostate surgery is considered an ambulatory procedure because you enter the hospital the day of your surgery rather than the night before for preparation. Now patients do the preparation procedures themselves at home.

Preoperative Fasting

For the day before your surgery, you will not be allowed to consume anything except clear liquids—and you should have plenty of them. Clear liquid means liquid you can see through, including water, broth, or tea without milk, and any clear, unpulpy fruit juices except orange, grapefruit, and tomato. Milk products and carbonated beverages are prohibited. After midnight before the day of surgery, you cannot eat or drink anything, not even water. Also, you must refrain from smoking or drinking alcohol during this time. Only a sip of water can be used to take medications.

Self-Administered Enema

A self-administered Fleet enema can be done the night before surgery to clean out your rectum. An enema is the insertion of fluid through the anus into your rectum to flush out fecal matter. Some urologists may prefer that you drink a saline solution, which induces diarrhea in order to clean out your bowel. Some may ask that you do both. Some hospitals may want you to take a half bottle of magnesium citrate in the morning of the day before surgery. Enemas are available without prescription from pharmacies.

What to Pack

You will need your own personal items such as a toothbrush and shaving gear, but you probably won't need your own pajamas and robe unless you absolutely cannot tolerate wearing hospital issue. Bring some loose-fitting trousers for the trip home and possibly a pillow to sit on if you will be sitting in a car for any length of time.

Ask family members to hang on to your eyeglasses, cane, and your assistive device if you have one. A hearing aid can be worn during surgery, but contact lenses cannot.

Bring your insurance card with you as well as a check or credit card to pay for rental of a television or telephone.

The Day of Surgery

The day you come in for surgery, the entire surgical procedure should be explained again, usually by the nursing staff and your urologist. You should expect to be questioned about any concerns you may have and how well you understand the follow-up procedures, such as coping with the catheter and whether or not you have been practicing the Kegel exercises, which strengthen the urinary sphincter muscle. See Chapter 17 for information about Kegels.

If you can have your surgery scheduled as the first one of the day, you will probably have your procedure done on time. Naturally, if there are others before you in the operating room, then the time is only an estimate. If there is a complication or reason for delay with another patient, your waiting period will lengthen. Generally, your spouse or friend can stay with you until you are called for surgery.

You may be given an antibiotic but probably not a tranquilizer, despite any anxiety you may be feeling.

Meeting the Anesthesiologist

Your anesthesiologist will talk with you about his or her role. (This is usually just before surgery, but in some hospitals you may meet this physician during your preoperative testing period.) Expect to be questioned about reactions you may have had to anesthesia in the past. Ask what kind of anesthesia will be used, how it will affect you, and any aftereffects you can expect. Be forthcoming about *all* drugs you are taking. As drugs and techniques have improved, the risks of anesthesia have decreased dramatically.

Although general anesthesia, which puts you to sleep, is still used in some prostatectomies, most prostate surgery is done with an epidural, a regional anesthesia that makes you numb from the waist down. Epidural anesthesia is inserted through a tiny plastic tube between two vertebrae in your back. The catheter through which the epidural anesthesia is administered is left in after surgery so that pain medications can be administered directly to the site. This is helpful for postoperative pain management. The anesthetic soaks into the area outside the dura, the membrane lining the spinal cord. The area below the insertion becomes numb. The epidural is usually accompanied by an IV medication to make you drowsy or sedated so that you drift off to sleep during the operation, but you will not be unconscious as with general anesthesia.

The anesthesiologist stays with you throughout the operation to monitor your blood pressure and heart rhythm, and to talk with you if you are awake. If you have general anesthesia you will be completely unconscious, and a tube inserted into your throat and connected to a respirator will control your breathing for you.

In the Operating Room

The nurses and the anesthesiologist get you ready for surgery. Your abdomen will be painted with antiseptic and your pubic hair shaved. Pneumatic boots will be put on your legs to help maintain good circulation while you are asleep and to minimize the chance of developing a blood clot in your legs, which is known as deep venous thrombosis (DVT). Operating rooms are necessarily chilly in order to keep the multigowned surgeons and staff cool during the lengthy time in an enclosed area with high-powered lights and other equipment. You will be covered with sterile drapes and a warm blanket.

Because anesthesia will interfere with your body's ability to regulate its own temperature, it is important that you be kept warm. A drop in body temperature inhibits defenses against germs, decreases the blood flow to the skin, and lowers the supply of oxygen necessary to fight infection. Cold also interferes with blood clotting.

A urethral catheter will be inserted through the urethra into your bladder to drain off urine that collects in your bladder during surgery. During this time, the anesthetic will begin to make you relax, your surgeon may come in and talk with you. Surgery takes about $2^1/_2$ to 3 hours.

After Surgery

When you leave the operating room, you will be taken to the recovery room while the anesthesia wears off. Your blood pressure will be checked frequently by the nurses monitoring you until your vital signs are stabilized. You may be given a painkiller such as ketorolac tromethamine (Toradol), and an IV will be feeding you salt water mixed with glucose. You may be in the recovery room for 3 to 4 hours or more.

From the time you enter the hospital to the time you leave the recovery room and go to your own room, an entire day will have passed. Your family can wait for you in the waiting room or in your hospital room, but they are generally not allowed into hospital recovery rooms.

Following surgery, you will probably be in the hospital for 3 to 5 days. You will not be in bed the entire time. In fact, your surgeon may want you up and walking by the next day. Compression boots may be kept on your legs when you are lying in bed to keep the circulation to your lower extremities normal. A urethral catheter will continue to drain urine from your bladder. The first day, you will be fed intravenously until your system recovers from the anesthesia. Thirst will be quenched by sucking on ice cubes. Most patients begin a regular diet a day or two after surgery.

Controlling Pain

Pain can be moderate to severe for the first 24 to 48 hours after a radical prostatectomy, gradually easing off, perhaps with the help of Toradol or other common analgesics, or the patient-controlled analgesia system if it is available at your hospital. All men respond differently to pain and there are many physiological reasons for the degree of pain. There is real physical pain and soreness from the trauma of surgery. There is a degree of anxiety and fear. These factors combine to alter pain perception. Always acknowledge your pain. Don't be too stoic.

In modern medical centers, patients now manage their own pain medications with the PCA system—patient-controlled analgesia. Pain medications are delivered from a nearby machine attached to your epidural tube. You can press the button and get more pain relief if you need it, but the PCA system is regulated to release a certain amount of pain medication per hour so there is no fear of overdosing. The system is computer operated, so if you are getting no pain relief, ask the hospital staff to check the computer setting.

You may feel pain from your incision as it heals. You may also find it painful to sit up, cough, or sneeze for a few days. Anything that calls on your abdominal muscles, which are understandably stressed, could make you feel sore. Several layers of your abdomen—muscle, fat, skin—around your incision must heal.

After prostate surgery it is common to feel some bladder pressure, like an urgent need to urinate. This is because of the catheter in your bladder. When this pressure is intense, you may feel spasms in your bladder. Let your nurse and doctor know about this. There are special medications for this problem if spasms occur frequently or become severe.

Caring for Your Incision

For the first few days, great care will be taken around the wound site to avoid contamination and infection. The incision is usually about 8 inches long, from your navel to pubis. Once the wound has begun to heal, usually after about 2 days, the dressing can be left off. As the incision heals, a hard ridge will form, but this will gradually recede over the next few months.

You may have two drains, one on each side of the pelvis to drain the lymph node dissection site. The drains are small plastic tubes connected to a collection device to monitor the amount of drainage of lymphatic fluid. Once the drainage decreases enough, your doctor will remove the drains. Once they are out, the area where they were may still feel sore for a few days.

If your incision is stapled shut, the staples will be removed—with a staple remover—usually by the seventh day after surgery. If the incision is sealed with Steri Strips, these fall off on their own after about 2 weeks. Once you get home, you can bathe or shower normally, but wash around your wound gently with mild, unscented soap, and pat it dry. It is normal for the skin around your incision to be slightly red. This redness gradually fades. Call your doctor if you notice severe redness, swelling, or oozing. Sometimes a warm heating pad can relieve pain around the incision.

Activity and Exercise

Unless surgery was extensive or complicated, most surgeons want their patients up and walking by the day after surgery. You may feel wobbly and you will be attached to tubes, so the nurses or one of your visitors can help you walk short distances, for instance, down the corridor or to the hospital lounge.

After open abdominal surgery, take special care not to put pressure on your abdominal muscles until your incision is well healed. Regular activity and walking are good, but you should not do anything strenuous for about 6 weeks. There may be limitations on lifting anything that will call on your abdominal muscles. Ask your surgeon for detailed instructions. If he or she says no heavy lifting, ask what is considered heavy. Some say nothing heavier than a phone book. Obviously you won't do situps or pushups, but you might bend down to pick up the newspaper from your doorstep and pull your abdominal muscles. Ask about the best techniques for getting up from a bed or chair, bending, lifting, reaching, and stretching.

Too much activity can cause problems with your catheter. Remember never to pull on the catheter. It is held in place inside your bladder by an inflated balloon and can disrupt the urethral anastomosis if pulled.

Once you get home, you may find that you tire easily, but your energy will return gradually. Try to relax and take it easy. You may need to lie down in the afternoon. Climb stairs very slowly and rest when you are tired. If you are an active person, you will generally recover quickly. If you are a couch potato, it may take longer.

Eating and Drinking

By the second day, you should be able to eat and drink normally. Generally, a well-balanced diet helps the healing process, but because the wall of your rectum will be tender for a while and you may also be dehydrated, you can become constipated. If you push or strain to have a bowel movement, you may feel pain. Your doctor may advise using a stool softener and laxative to ease this condition. Drink lots of fluids.

Functioning with a Catheter

A catheter will extend from your penis for up to 3 weeks so that the urine will drain without putting any stress on your rebuilt lower urinary tract. A balloon attached to the other end of the catheter is inside your bladder to hold it in place. It will take about 3 weeks for the anastomosis—the newly created connection of your urethra to your bladder neck—to heal.

The hospital staff will teach you how to manage the catheter so that the urine can drain into a receptacle. In fact, most hospitals cannot discharge you until they are confident that you can operate the receptacles that collect the urine. A larger overnight urinary bag is usually fastened to the bed; a smaller leg bag is strapped around your thigh and the catheter is attached to it. You can wear trousers with the leg bag so that you can go out without having to carry the larger bag. The large capacity of the overnight bag allows you to sleep through the night without having to empty it.

Postoperative Depression

After the keyed-up adrenaline generated before the surgery, some men feel an emotional crash after surgery. This is natural. Facing radical prostate surgery is unlike other surgery preceded by obvious symptoms such as heart pain or a broken limb. Many men are otherwise perfectly healthy, and having to face the prospect and the aftermath of major surgery may change their outlook on life forever.

Because prostate cancer often happens in middle age, it may coincide with midlife crisis. You have worked hard and struggled through the early years, raised your family, established your career, and now that you have reached the point where your life should be smooth sailing, cancer has hit you like a ton of bricks. You may ask yourself, "What is there to live for?" It is normal to be depressed following surgery. The best way to cope with depression is to just let yourself feel it, talk about it if you can, go through it, and move on.

Be forthcoming about your feelings with your doctor. If your doctor is thoughtful and has good insight into your personality and lifestyle, as well as a sense of your relationship with your spouse or partner if you have one, he or she can help you. By giving you specific, doable, short-term goals, a physician can help you through the process one step at a time. For example, the first goal will be to see the pathology report to find out if the cancer is contained within the prostate gland. Then you can plan for the removal of the catheter and begin the Kegel exercises or techniques to strengthen your external sphincter muscle. Plan activities for the weeks ahead—going back to work, getting your checkups, monitoring your PSA—and gradually, one step at a time, your spirits will be restored.

Before You Go Home: A Checklist

It will take you a couple of months to feel normal again, so before you leave the hospital be sure to get written instructions about caring for your incision at home, managing the catheter, and performing other follow-up care. It's better to ask questions and take some notes yourself so that you can refer to them at home. Be sure you know about the following:

- What to do if the catheter falls out
- Pain medications to take if you need them
- Signs of infection and what to watch for
- When you can take a shower or tub bath
- When to see the doctors for follow-up visits
- When to call the doctor if something is bothering you

- How often to change the dressing on your incision
- Clothing to wear to cover the catheter bag
- When to begin normal physical activity and exercising
- What to eat or not eat while recovering
- What to expect from urine and bowel function; how to identify a problem
- Home health care nurses: Will you need them and what do they provide?
- Where to get professional help for your emotional ups and downs
- How to find the nearest support group

11

External Beam Radiation Therapy

Radiation therapy, like surgery, is local treatment—it treats only the area it touches. Where surgery cuts out and removes the prostate and the tumor, radiation kills the prostate cancer cells by altering the deoxyribonucleic acid (DNA) and scarifying the blood vessels so blood cannot flow and feed the cancer.

Radiation therapy, which has been in use in one form or another for over a century, uses approximately 500 to 1,000 times more energy than what is used with regular diagnostic X-rays. This high dosage from high-energy equipment penetrates the tissue as it passes through the body and is absorbed. It radiates all the cells in its path—good and bad—so they cannot grow and multiply. Radiation damages cellular DNA. Cancer cells are more sensitive than normal cells to radiation because they are dividing rapidly, so treatment prevents the cancer cells from multiplying.

Radiation is also known as irradiation or radiotherapy, and it can be delivered externally or internally. External beam radiation is most commonly used, but the implantation of radioactive seeds—brachytherapy—into the prostate is becoming more popular as treatment techniques improve.

The side effects of radiation therapy have a lasting impact on lifestyle, so it is important that you understand what they are and how you can correct them or live with them. Despite sophisticated high-precision techniques, it is impossible to prevent some damage to the blood vessels around the prostate. Damage can also occur to the neurovascular bundles. When these vessels become scarified, blood cannot flow into the penis, and nerve damage can result, causing erectile dysfunction or impotence in 30 to 40 percent of patients.

Although radiation therapy is used for all stages of prostate cancer, it has the best chance of curing low-volume prostate cancers—those diagnosed as T1 or T2 tumors. More advanced cancer is sometimes treated with radiation, but then it is meant to alleviate bone pain or treat symptoms such as obstruction of the urethra. It is common to use radiation as palliative therapy for patients who have pain from bone metastases.

Some radiation oncologists believe radiation therapy is effective in any cancer that has not yet metastasized, no matter how big the tumor. For example, a patient with a T3 tumor would not be a good candidate for surgery, but he may be a reasonable candidate for radiation therapy. When prostate cancer spreads, it often causes obstruction in the bladder area, resulting in difficult urination or damage to kidney function. Radiation therapy can often get to those areas and relieve the obstructive symptoms, which is one of the reasons it is important in treating more advanced prostate cancer.

Although there is still a wide disparity of opinions among radiation oncologists and urologists, most would agree that any man who has a life expectancy under 10 years and has other medical problems would be a better candidate for radiation therapy because surgery might be too risky.

Some look at it this way: Assuming a T1 or T2 cancer, surgery may be a good choice if the PSA is under 10, when there is an 80 to 90 percent cure potential. If it is over 10, either surgery or radiation could be effective. When the PSA is over 20, radiation is usually a better choice than surgery because the chance of metastasis is much greater with higher PSA values. For example, radiation therapy would not necessarily get all cancer cells, but it would get many and also avoid the risks of surgery.

We need more long-term studies before we can know for sure how effective radiation treatment will be against prostate cancer. As of 1997, radiation therapy compared favorably with surgery for treating early-stage cancer in studies with a minimum five-year follow-up. More than half the men with T1 or T2 tumors and low Gleason scores appear to be cured with external beam radiation therapy. The results are not as clear with bulkier tumors, which have a lower chance of cure. Radiation in combination with hormone therapy can add additional survival time by theoretically downstaging the tumor.

Despite the lack of long-term studies to demonstrate that radiation is as good as or better than surgery for curing prostate cancer, there has been an increased interest in radiation therapy because of greater media attention in the 1990s. Many high-profile men have had this treatment and have written about it in books and magazines. There is also the matter of the technology itself, which has improved dramatically in recent years with increasing numbers of hospitals installing the kind of sophisticated machinery and computer-assisted equipment needed to deliver more precise treatment.

How It Works

External beam radiation has been used in the treatment of prostate cancer since the 1950s. Cobalt, a radioactive isotope, was used in the earliest treatments, but currently many centers utilize the high-energy radiation produced by a linear accelerator that generates and directs the beams–X-rays, gamma rays, or electrons–to the target area. Radiation treatment is delivered and tailored to each individual case.

Radiation is measured much the way watts of electricity are measured. The unit of measurement for radiation is the gray (Gy). The old measurement unit was a rad, and some physicians and technologists still use this measurement term. One Gy equals 100 rads. A typical daily dose of radiation to treat prostate cancer is 1.8 to 2.0 Gy, or 180 to 200 rads.

Naturally, the higher the dose of radiation, the better the chance of killing the cancer, but there are limits to the amount of radiation that can be safely delivered to the human body. Although your body can tolerate large amounts of radiation, it cannot tolerate it all at once. It was believed until the mid-1980s that the maximum safe dose for prostate cancer was 70 Gy (7,000 rads) administered in small doses over a period of weeks. To prevent harm to other organs, such as the bladder and rectum, the 70 Gy of radiation was given in small daily doses, 5 days a week, for 6 to 9 weeks. With more sophisticated technology, such as high-quality CAT and MRI scans and computer-assisted planning modules, higher doses can now be delivered safely.

Three-Dimensional (3D) Conformal Technique

Until the end of the 1980s, conventional two-dimensional radiation (still in use in many centers) provided a dose of only 7,000 rads in the four-field technique with beams aimed at the front, back, left, and right sides of the patient. A wide area of the pelvis was irradiated, including the rectum and bladder, in an attempt to treat all of the cancer.

The advent of computer technology helped radiation therapists move from simple two-dimensional X-rays to three-dimensional–3D–conformal treatment. This profound improvement in the accuracy of the treatment means it is no longer necessary to irradiate such a wide area around the prostate. *Conformal* means the radiation field "conforms" to the shape of the prostate and the radiation beam can be aimed in an oblique angle to hit the target more precisely without doing as much damage to the other adjacent organs. This technique requires more sophisticated computer software, but this equipment is becoming more widely available in medical centers.

By the mid-1990s, experts seemed to agree that as much as 80 Gy (8,000 rads) could be delivered safely. The new technology allows penetration of the target area with very little radiation touching the bladder and rectum. Beams can be focused on the prostate and seminal vesicles with only an inch or so of margin. Thus, by limiting the area around the prostate that could be exposed to injury, increased radiation doses can be applied directly to the cancer more safely. Still, not all physicians are willing to use higher doses until more long-term studies have been completed, which has added to the controversy in prostate cancer treatment.

Simulation: Planning Treatment

Radiation treatment requires about a week of preparation. First, one or two consultations with the radiation oncologist are needed before you begin. Then there are several days of preparation with your treatment team to be sure the radiation is delivered as precisely as possible. Your radiation oncologist will review your medical history, pathology reports, medical records, bone scan, CAT or MRI scans, and talk with you about your particular treatment. There may be some additional testing such as blood tests or X-rays. Your actual treatment can begin within a week or two from your initial consultation.

Accuracy in delivering radiation to the cancer cells is of critical importance in order to avoid injury to the bladder and rectum. Thus, a sort of dress rehearsal known as simulation is needed. The treatment center's physicist and dosimetrist can study your prostate and the surrounding area while you are in the CAT scanner. The computer then calculates the location of all the other organs on the CAT scan. They carefully map out a plan for sending the radiation beam directed at your tumor with as little damage to the bladder and rectum as possible.

The simulation for this technique is the same as for conventional treatment. Your pelvic area is measured and marked first with marking pens and then finally with tiny tattoos to guide the technicians in aiming the radiation beam at your prostate.

Your prostate and surrounding organs are uniquely your own are not exactly the same size and shape as any other man's, so your treatment must be tailored to fit you just like a good suit. The bladder and rectum are not static organs. They live and breathe with you, so their exact location may change by a fraction of an inch in different positions. Careful planning and a custom-made plastic body cast or cradle hold you precisely in place during treatment. Lead blocks may also be custom designed to protect nearby healthy tissue from radiation.

All this sophisticated preparation will determine not only at what angle the beam should enter your body, but what shape the beam should be. Several beams will be entering your body to intersect at the target area. The ability to plan treatment from the perspective of the beam is known as beam's eye view. The beam entry is controlled and the tumor is viewed from all angles. This technique reduces complications, especially rectal bleeding and irritative voiding symptoms.

The Treatment Process

Radiation treatment for prostate cancer is given daily from Monday through Friday for 6 to 9 weeks. Daily treatments are administered by the radiation therapists. You should be in the treatment center no more than an hour from the time you sign in, change into a dressing gown, and receive your treatment.

For the treatment itself, you lie on your back or on your stomach. The technicians get you into place on the treatment table. They return to the control room and watch you through a window, as well as through a closed-circuit television, while they administer the treatment. The radiation machine revolves around you and the radiation is sent into your prostate area for only a few seconds, although you may be in position for 5 minutes or more. You won't feel a thing.

It is always best to lead as normal a life as possible during the weeks of treatment. However, radiation can make you tired, it can irritate your skin, and it may cause some gastrointestinal problems, so don't expect to function at full capacity. Rest when you need to. If you can schedule treatment for mornings or late in the afternoon, you can continue your work with little interruption to your day. If you miss a treatment because of a holiday or bad weather, another day can be added to your treatment schedule, but treatments should not be missed often. A 5-day delay should not interfere with therapy, but more than that can.

Many patients who live far away move near the radiation treatment center for the entire 2 months so that they can avoid the long commute. If you relocate, be sure to ask the patient services representative about discounted housing that may be available through the hospital.

Short-Term Side Effects

Side effects from radiation treatment don't normally show up until you have been in treatment for about 2 weeks. Then the cumulative dose of radiation may begin to cause minor problems such as inflammation of the prostate, skin irritation, more frequent urination and possibly burning on urination, diarrhea, and fatigue. Once treatment ends, these side effects gradually diminish after a few weeks.

•   **Skin Irritation**.   After a week or two, your pelvic area may swell and your skin may become slightly pink or a deep red and itchy in the treated area. The intensity varies with each individual and skin type. Avoid irritation by wearing clothes that will not rub against your skin. Boxer shorts and loose-fitting trousers are a good idea.

To take care of your skin during radiation treatment, use clear warm water instead of soap and creams in the treatment areas. Pat yourself dry and don't rub. If you are itchy, ask your therapist about special creams that will not interfere with treatment. Prescription creams or a light sprinkling of cornstarch may help. Avoid heavy lotions. They may leave a coating on your skin that can interfere with your treatment and cause further irritation.

•   **Urinary Changes**.   After the first 2 weeks, you may urinate more often, especially during the night, and you may also feel a mild burning sensation if your prostate is inflamed from the radiation. However, these symptoms usually level off after about 3 weeks of radiation and do not get any worse. Long-term urinary complications are rare, but your bladder function may not be exactly as it was before treatment. You may feel a sense of urgency or feel the need to urinate more often. Perhaps 1 in every 100 patients will have some form of urinary incontinence.

• **Bowel Problems.** Diarrhea was a common side effect with the older radiation technology because more of the pelvis was irradiated during the treatment, exposing the bowel to potential injury. This problem is less common now. The back of the rectum is about an inch behind the prostate and this part of the rectum will receive as much radiation as the prostate. There may be irritation during bowel movements, as well as diarrhea, and an increase in the number of bowel movements. These symptoms will subside 2 to 3 weeks after radiation treatments.

About 5 percent of treated men may experience rectal bleeding after radiation if the rectum was particularly sensitive to the radiation. It usually occurs only during bowel movements because of the pressure of stool passing through the rectum and increased irritation of hemorrhoidal tissue. This type of bleeding usually goes away by itself within 1 to 5 years. If the bleeding is severe, you may need a temporary colostomy to divert the colon and the fecal stream to a bag outside your body until the rectum heals. Generally, the rectum will heal and the colostomy can be reversed. The chance of this complication is less than 1 percent.

Long-Term Side Effects

Whereas the urinary and bowel symptoms will generally subside quickly, there are longer-term side effects, such as impotence, that can progress anywhere from 6 months to 2 years after the end of radiation treatment. Impotence caused by radiation is permanent, with the chance of occurrence increasing with age. Impotence is caused by the effects of radiation as well as the natural effects of aging. After 1 year, about 10 percent of irradiated men are impotent. Overall, there is a 30 to 40 percent chance of impotence after radiation.

Radiation scarifies the blood vessels that carry blood to the penis for an erection and may damage the neurovascular bundles. But impotence does not decrease your sexual desire (libido) or your ability to achieve orgasm. Impotence does not mean that you will no longer have a sex life. It simply means that you will have to adapt to new ways of achieving an erection. It is very important to discuss this matter openly with your physician as well as your spouse or intimate partner so that you can learn how to deal with it. There are medications and mechanical devices, as well as surgical prostheses, to help men with erectile dysfunction. See Chapter 18 for ways to restore potency.

A small amount of "scatter radiation," something like nuclear fallout, may reach your testicles, and there can be some damage to sperm. Although most men who undergo prostate treatment are past their parenting years, it would be wise to bank some sperm before treatment if you are planning to father a child.

There is no evidence that radiation will increase the risk of any other cancer such as lymphoma.

Combination Therapies

In some cases, external beam radiation therapy may be combined with other therapy, such as hormonal therapy, so-called salvage surgery, or brachytherapy, an internal radiation therapy described in the next chapter. Brachytherapy, involving the implantation of radioactive seeds into the prostate, is generally used for early-stage and small tumors. However, combining the implantation with external beam therapy is occasionally used for a more locally advanced tumor to increase the level of radiation that can be delivered to the site of the cancer. Sometimes seeds are implanted before or after a course of external beam radiation therapy to act as a booster. This procedure may be used with an aggressive cancer, but it is not generally used when the cancer has metastasized.

Neoadjuvant Hormone Therapy

In some cases, 2 or 3 months of hormonal therapy may precede treatment with radiation. The goal is to shrink or downstage the tumor and reduce the field of radiation. With a smaller target, less surrounding tissue will be damaged from radiation. There are studies underway to determine if this strategy delays recurrence of the disease. In theory it is very appealing, but we won't know the answer for several years.

Radiation and "Salvage" Surgery

Prostate surgery for persistent prostate cancer after radiation therapy is sometimes called "salvage" surgery, and most physicians consider this procedure ineffective in removing residual disease except in rare cases. About half the men who have this surgery after the failure of radiation therapy become incontinent of urine and nearly all of them become impotent. However, because as many as 20 percent of men may appear to be cured after such treatment, some are willing to take the risk if they are in good general health.

Salvage surgery is difficult because once the prostate has been irradiated there is considerable scar tissue. The normal anatomic planes of dissection are often lost and surgery can potentially injure the rectum, bladder, and surrounding blood vessels.

A 50-year-old investment banker had a PSA of 7.4 and the DRE revealed evidence of a large tumor involving both lobes of the prostate. He was diagnosed with inoperable cancer because of stage, tumor size, and Gleason score, and advised to have neoadjuvant hormonal therapy to shrink the tumor followed by a course of 3D conformal radiation therapy. Thinking ahead, this man wanted to know his options if cancer recurred after radiation. Would his doctor try salvage surgery to remove the prostate? This course does not normally accomplish much, especially since the radiated prostate is all scar tissue and often falls apart when it is dissected. However, because this man was otherwise healthy and relatively young, he and his physician considered salvage surgery an acceptable option if the radiation therapy proved ineffective.

Follow-Up Care

When radiation therapy is completed, expect to have a routine checkup with your radiation oncologist within 2 months, and then alternate checkups between your radiation oncologist and urologist every 3 months for 2 years, then every 6 months for 5 years. This follow-up may include a periodic transrectal sonogram of the prostate to look for residual disease.

If cancer has been destroyed by radiation therapy, your PSA should gradually fall to low levels within the year following therapy. If it drops to less than 1.0, it is likely the cancer is gone. If the level is above 2 after a year, it is likely there is still some cancer present. If the PSA rises after treatment, then bone and CAT scans can determine if there is any metastatic disease present.

The Radiation Treatment Team

Teaching hospitals and comprehensive cancer centers often provide the best radiation therapy because they treat a large volume of patients, attract experienced physicians, and use up-to-date equipment. You will want to know that there is a CAT scanner available and a physicist on staff to handle problems that may arise with the equipment. Radiation oncology centers and hospital departments of nuclear medicine must be approved by federal and state nuclear regulatory agencies. Most important, you'll want to know how many cases of prostate cancer are treated at a particular facility each year.

You can find a radiation oncologist and radiation treatment center by calling the American Cancer Society, the National Cancer Institute, or the American College of Radiology. Libraries, cancer hotlines, and support groups are also good sources of information. For more information on radiation treatment for prostate cancer, call the National Cancer Institute for their free booklet, *Radiation Therapy and You.*

Radiation Oncologists

A radiation oncologist (sometimes called a radiation therapist or radiotherapist) is a physician who is specially trained in treating cancer with radiation therapy, which is not the same as a radiologist who specializes in the diagnosis of disease using X-rays. The radiation oncologist will probably be recommended by your urologist, but do not accept a radiation oncologist with whom you do not feet comfortable. In large treatment centers there will be more than one with whom you can talk. Expect your radiation oncologist to consult with you and your urologist, review your medical reports, and examine you thoroughly before administering your radiotherapy.

Ask questions about the physician's background and experience in treating prostate cancer. You'll want to know about his or her board certification and number of years treating prostate cancer. Will the radiation oncologist personally supervise your treatment or will technicians handle the daily routine? If you are dealing with technicians, expect your radiation oncologist to talk with you and examine you at least once a week during your course of treatment. Be sure to ask about the side effects. Also ask about the chance of receiving this treatment again in the future if the cancer metastasizes. How often will you be able to talk with this doctor? Can you call with questions?

The Technicians

The other health care professionals directly involved in your treatment include the therapist, and behind the scenes, the physicist and dosimetrist. Therapists are state-licensed technicians with 2 to 4 years of special training. They generally administer your daily treatment following the guidelines set up by your radiation oncologist. The therapist will position you for each treatment and direct the linear accelerator to deliver your precise dose of radiation.

Radiation physicists and dosimetrists are the planners of your treatment. With the radiation oncologist, the physicist designs and develops the best possible therapy for cure according to your individual case. The physicist is also in charge of quality control for the equipment. The dosimetrist calculates the exact amount of radiation you will get.

The Cost of Radiation Therapy

A complete program of radiation therapy for prostate cancer can cost tens of thousands of dollars in a large medical center, including treatment planning and 30 to 45 treatments. There will be professional charges from the people who give you the treatment as well as hospital charges for delivery of the services. Most medical insurance covers these charges. Medicare covers 80 percent of the cost and Medicaid covers it all. If you are insured by a health maintenance organization, be sure you understand the rules governing radiation treatment.

Also, keep in mind that if you are traveling from a distance to get treatment, or you are actually living in a different city during the weeks of treatment, those expenses may be covered by your insurance. (They are also deductible as a medical expense on your income tax.) Some treatment centers have access to reduced-cost hotels in the area or other moderately priced temporary housing.

Brachytherapy (see Chapter 12) is less costly than external beam radiation and requires only a single procedure rather than weeks of treatment, which could be an advantage for those who live far from a radiation facility.

12

Brachytherapy (Interstitial Radiation)

Brachytherapy is a form of radiation therapy in which radioactive isotopes are surgically implanted directly into the prostate. Brachy means "short distance," and the radiation from the isotopes, or seeds as they are called, works in the immediate area over a continuous period—24 hours a day—compared with the daily bursts of radiation used in external beam treatment. This type of radiation is sometimes called interstitial (in the narrow spaces) radiation therapy.

As local control rates after external beam appear to be dose dependent, it is theorized that higher doses of radiation can be given directly to the prostate if the isotopes are accurately placed through a needle into the prostate. In the past, there was no technique to assure this accurate placement. An open surgical technique did not allow the brachytherapist to clearly visualize placement of needles and seeds during the procedure. Few seed implantations with open surgery had a homogeneous distribution within the prostate. In retrospect, it was not possible to determine whether the seeds were placed in the exact area where the cancer was located. With very early cancer, this technique seemed to provide reasonably good local control only in men who had an adequate radiation dose. But what was adequate?

Because results of those early brachytherapy treatments were inferior to most external beam treatment regimens, the procedure was abandoned until better seed placement techniques were developed. The same technology that made 3D conformal therapy possible now makes better seed placement possible. In most cases, treatment can be given as a single outpatient visit and men can return to "normal" life in a few days. Risk of urinary incontinence is extremely low and the expectation of maintaining potency is high.

Seed implantation is now used as a stand-alone treatment or as a boost treatment following moderate doses of external beam radiation therapy. Selecting patients into a low-risk group suitable for seed implementation alone and a high-risk group for combination seed therapy and external beam therapy is difficult. Again, we must wait for results of long-term studies.

For some patients brachytherapy is considered an attractive alternative to surgery and external beam radiation. Some clinical series suggest that the progression-free survival rate for 5 years may be superior to external beam therapy and equal to radical surgery for patients with a PSA less than 10.

The radioactive seeds are smaller than sesame seeds and they emit radiation over a long period of time. In the past, radioactive gold was used, but now palladium and iodine are used. Seeds of palladium 103 provide over 12,000 rads or 120 Gy, and seeds of iodine 125 provide over 10,000 rads or 100 Gy. Palladium treats for 20 days, whereas iodine treats for more than 60 days. When the radiation is used up, the seeds become dormant and remain in the prostate.

Some data suggest that iodine appears to be preferred in treating slow-growing tumors typical of many prostate cancer patients. However, this issue is controversial because clinical studies have yet to confirm its effectiveness. At present, iodine is used in most centers for low- and moderate-grade cancers with Gleason scores of 2 to 6, and palladium is used for more poorly differentiated cancers with Gleason scores of 8 to 10. With a Gleason score of 6 or 7, either isotope can be used.

Disadvantages are that we have no long-term studies that can lead us to believe conclusively that seed implant therapy is any better than watchful waiting, surgery, or external beam radiation. We do know it may delay the recurrence of prostate cancer even though it may not cure it. There are also no long-term studies to tell us whether leaving seeds in the prostate causes any damage to other organs. About 10 to 30 percent of men are left impotent from brachytherapy compared with 30 to 40 percent with external beam radiation.

The Procedure

The radioactive seeds are implanted in the prostate by a urologist and a radiation oncologist in the hospital while you are under spinal or general anesthesia. The urologist and radiation oncologist work together on this procedure with the guidance of the physicist. The same sophisticated computer and scanning techniques that make 3D conformal radiation so precise are also used to place the seeds with great precision.

The implantation is generally an outpatient procedure performed with regional anesthesia to numb the patient from the waist down. Various templates are positioned against the perineum to guide the needles along the right path. Most of these procedures are done with needles inserted through the perineal area between the scrotum and the anus. Guided by ultrasound, the physician can accurately place the seeds through a thin tube (catheter). When the tube is withdrawn, the seeds are left in place.

The number of seeds implanted depends on the size of the prostate and the extent of the cancer, but on average there may be 50 to 100 seeds implanted in the entire prostate, although 200 is not uncommon. The seeds are implanted one at a time while the surgeon monitors the ultrasound screen. Sometimes seeds are implanted in the seminal vesicles as well.

Who Is a Candidate for Brachytherapy?

The ideal candidate for permanent seed implantation is a man with an intact prostate with a volume of less than 2 ounces. Such a patient would be less likely to suffer serious rectal or urinary complications as side effects.

Internal radiation is generally recommended for a small localized tumor and a PSA of less than 10. If cancer cells were found in more than one lobe of the prostate during needle biopsy or anywhere near the seminal vesicles, then brachytherapy would not be as effective.

Brachytherapy alone appears to be suitable for patients who have a high chance that their cancer is still confined to the prostate. Those with a substantial chance of extracapsular disease (cancer that appears to have broken out of the prostate) may be more suitable for combination therapy of external beam radiation and brachytherapy. Some patients even consider having hormonal therapy before brachytherapy in an attempt to make the tumor smaller or downstage it. This therapy can be done 3 months or more before brachytherapy. Long-term studies of this treatment are in progress, but we will not have results for several years.

In general, men with T1 or T2-A cancer, a PSA of less than 10, and a Gleason score of between 2 and 6 are reasonable candidates for brachytherapy alone. Those with T2-B or T2-C disease, a PSA greater than 10, or a Gleason score from 7 to 10 should consider combined therapy. Men with cancer staged at T3, or with positive lymph nodes, would not be good candidates for permanent seed implantation.

Treatment Planning

Today we can use transrectal ultrasound (TRUS) and computer dosimetry to place seeds accurately, and we hope to significantly improve the cancer survival results. With TRUS allowing the therapist to visualize the needle placement and the computer reconstructing the prostate in three dimensions, before implantation we can create an ideal model for treatment planning. We can determine the amount of radiation needed for a particular individual and use sophisticated systems of seed placement customized to each patient's prostate size and shape. The needles are inserted through the perineum, the area between the scrotum and rectum, guided by the ultrasound. The physician can plan placement of needles that will transport the seeds as well as the type of activity and number of seeds to be planted. The amount of radiation needed to optimize the dose to the prostate and minimize the dose to the bladder and rectum is calculated with computer dosimetry.

Treatment Team

A dedicated team consisting of a urologist, radiation oncologist, and physicist can perform the technique successfully. The procedure is done in the operating room while the patient is under anesthesia.

Permanent transperineal seed implantation is typically done as a single operative treatment using spinal anesthesia. There is no surgical incision, since needles are inserted through a template system directly into the perineum and directed to the predetermined targets under TRUS guidance. A typical implant requires from 50 to 100 seeds.

Following the operation, patients are usually given antibiotics, anti-inflammatory medications, and antispasmodic medications to prevent bladder pain and infection. Once the seeds are placed, they can be assessed with X-rays or a CAT scan. This type of assessment is usually done after the PSA evaluation and at 3-month intervals. In some cancer treatment centers, TRUS-guided biopsies of the prostate are performed several years or more after seed implantation to see whether residual prostate cancer exists.

Complications

Brachytherapy on an outpatient basis generally has minor complications. Most patients have some early symptoms of urinary frequency or urgency and outlet obstruction for 4 to 8 months after surgery. If urine is retained, temporary catheterization may be required. This symptom usually occurs in men who had urinary obstruction problems before treatment.

Complications of greater concern include proctitis, which occurs in from 2 to 12 percent of patients. This irritation of the rectum and anus from radiation causes diarrhea and blood in the stool, as well as pain in the rectum.

Although there are no long-term studies on the effectiveness of this therapy, researchers at Memorial Sloan-Kettering Cancer Center in New York found that it may be as effective as surgery for early-stage cancer. The study showed 60 percent of men treated with seeds had no evidence of cancer 5 years after treatment. A Seattle study found 97 percent of men free of cancer 4 years after brachytherapy. Although the early data look promising, we cannot be sure until long-term studies are completed.

The use of biopsy results or PSA progression to report treatment success is still controversial. However, rising PSA has been demonstrated to predict failure 2 to 5 years prior to clinical relapse. Therefore, the use of these parameters as end points may provide early clues for therapeutic effectiveness.

One man chose the treatment because of an unexpected circumstance. He was 67 and had a T1-C tumor with a Gleason score of 6. A bone scan showed no metastasis, but the CAT scan showed a kidney tumor. Surgery for the kidney tumor was done first, and the tumor was cancerous. Although the surgery was successful, the man went into a prolonged postoperative depression. When it was time to remove the prostate 6 months later, he said he could not face surgery again. Part of his depression may have had to do with his forced retirement and staying home alone while his wife worked. He agreed to brachytherapy. The therapy worked with few side effects. The man's emotional outlook has improved considerably.

Not all men come away from brachytherapy without complications, however, and it is important to have this procedure in a reputable facility where it is frequently performed. The first thing to ask the physician is how many brachytherapies he or she has performed.

Short-Term Side Effects of Implants

All those needle implants will leave the prostate and perineal area sore and you will feel this discomfort for about a week. A catheter placed in the bladder will control urination for a day or two. In general, the more potent the seeds, the more severe the side effects. Fewer side effects seem to occur in treatment centers where large numbers of these procedures are performed because the brachytherapists are more experienced.

• **Urinary Complications.** Most complications involve the urinary tract, causing increased frequency of urination, or discomfort or urgency. One in four men experience urinary problems such as urgency, frequency, burning, or blood in the urine. According to one study, side effects appeared to be permanent in about 7 percent of men. Incontinence occurred in 5 percent of patients, with stress incontinence being the problem in half of these patients. Stress incontinence is a small leakage of urine upon coughing or sneezing. In those who have had a TURP, however, the chance of incontinence increases to 6 to 20 percent.

• **Rectal Problems**. Pain, burning, frequency, urgency, and diarrhea are problems in about 5 percent of cases. These problems occur in greater numbers in men with large tumors.

• **Sexual Concerns**. Semen may appear red or brownish for a while because of blood, which is perfectly normal after this procedure. It will take several weeks or months to clear. The risk of impotence is 10 to 30 percent.

For several months the seeds will be radioactive. This is not a danger to you or to your spouse or partner. But in the first few months it would be wise to use a condom during intercourse in case a seed should accidentally come loose and be ejaculated.

The Nuclear Regulatory Commission has determined that constant close proximity by other people will not harm them. They will receive some radiation, however, so avoid having intercourse for the first several months after treatment with a woman who is or wants to be pregnant.

Questions to Ask About Radiation Therapy

• **What is the goal of this treatment?**
Radiation therapy can be used to try to cure the cancer, or it can be used as a way to slow it down. It is important for you to understand the goal.

• **How will the radiation be given and who will give it?**
External beam and brachytherapy are both complex and sophisticated procedures involving the skills of several people. With the external beam treatment, your radiation oncologist is in charge with the aid of technicians and the physicist. Brachytherapy, which combines radiation and surgery, involves your radiation oncologist working with your urologist and the physicist. If you have questions about brachytherapy, you will ask your urologist, and questions about external beam treatment will be addressed by your radiation oncologist.

• **How many prostate cancer patients are treated at this facility?**
It is always better to be treated where the staff has in-depth experience and treats many patients. Because accuracy is vital to successful treatment, it is wise to go to a facility that treats at least several cases a week similar to yours. Brachytherapy involves the skills of the urologist as well as the radiation oncologist and physicist; ask each doctor how many of these treatments he or she has done in the past. Keep in mind that brachytherapy has not been practiced very long, so you are more likely to find skilled practitioners in teaching hospitals. Studies have shown that success rates for brachytherapy are

higher where many of these procedures are performed. Accurate placement of the seeds requires special training and experience.

- **What side effects can I expect and what can I do about them?**

Everyone responds differently to treatment, but your doctor should explain all the possible side effects such as urinary or rectal problems, as well as the chances of impotence.

- **Can I choose the time of day when I get my treatment?**

External beam radiation can usually be scheduled at the most convenient time of day for you. Most people continue to work throughout the 6 to 9 weeks of treatment and it may be possible for you to have treatment early in the morning or late in the afternoon or even at lunchtime.

- **How up-to-date is your radiation equipment?**

The most recent and most sophisticated equipment has the capability of performing the 3D conformal radiation technique. A physicist and highly skilled technicians program and operate this equipment. More and more facilities have this technology, but some still operate with the older, less-advanced equipment. You should expect a thorough explanation before you decide to have treatment.

- **Who will treat me for any side effects?**

If you are having external beam radiation treatment, the radiation oncologist is responsible for your care during and after treatment. If you are having brachytherapy, the urologist and radiation oncologist are involved together in the treatment. It is a good idea to know who to call with a problem.

- **Will I have to wait long each day for treatment?**

In an efficiently operated radiation therapy facility, you should be in and out in less than an hour, which includes checking in, changing your clothes, receiving treatment, and getting dressed again.

PART FOUR

Treatment for Advanced Prostate Cancer

13

Hormonal Therapy for Metastatic Cancer

When Dr. Charles Huggins showed the world in 1941 that removing the testicles from a man with prostate cancer caused remission of the cancer, the world thought the treatment—orchiectomy—was a cure for prostate cancer. However, it was unknown at the time that some of the male hormones were also produced by the adrenal glands; years later, most of the patients had a recurrence of the cancer.

Huggins's remarkable research set the course for the manipulation of hormones as a treatment for prostate cancer. The very hormones that were responsible for the growth and development of a man or woman were also responsible for the growth and development of prostate cancer in men and breast cancer in women. With Huggins's discovery, drugs were developed to stop the production of testosterone just as orchiectomy did, and additional drugs were developed to deactivate the action of the hormones produced by the adrenal glands. Huggins shared the Nobel prize in 1966 with Clarence Hodges for their research involving the influence of hormones on prostate cancer.

Until recently, men receiving hormonal therapy had advanced stages of prostate cancer. Today, most men who receive hormonal therapy are those whose PSA levels are rising following surgery or radiation treatment. They may not have any symptoms of the disease, but because of the elevated PSA it is often necessary to restage the cancer with a bone scan and/or CAT (computerized axial tomography) scan. If the bone scan is negative, then it could mean the recurrence is only in the prostate area and the CAT scan will help to locate the site of the recurrence. If the cancer has reached the bones, it will show on the bone scan, and the CAT scan will not be necessary.

Hormonal therapy buys time, often many years or even a decade, but it does not cure prostate cancer. The goal of hormonal therapy is to slow the progression of the disease for as long as possible in order to extend survival and maintain quality of life. This approach is usually reserved for men whose tumors have spread beyond the prostate and for those who are unsuitable candidates for surgery or radiation. This therapy is also used as neoadjuvant therapy before surgery or radiation to shrink the tumor (downstaging). It is also used as an adjuvant therapy after surgery or radiation to slow the progression of cancer recurrence for as long as possible.

Some men's cancer may resist hormonal treatment sooner than others. One 77-year-old man whose cancer had already metastasized to his lymph nodes had many other things wrong with him. He had hypertension, heart disease that required bypass surgery, diverticulitis, and he was on several medications. Prostate surgery was not an option because of all of these medical conditions as well as his age. His only option was hormonal therapy or to do nothing. He chose to receive monthly hormone injections. Nevertheless, 7 years later, this man is still without symptoms of local or metastasized prostate cancer. He went into the hospital briefly this year, but that was because his heart condition deteriorated.

Most hormonal therapy is now provided with drugs that stop production or interfere with the action of androgens, even though the surgical removal of the testicles is easier to do and costs much less. The resistance of men to having their testicles removed is understandably strong, even in men who have little interest in sex. Hormonal therapy allows you to continue a normal life. Treatments generally are given by injection in your urologist's office monthly or quarterly, and sometimes with the addition of pills taken at home several times a day.

The most common side effect is loss of sex drive and sometimes hot flashes or some breast enlargement. (These hormones do not cause your voice to rise or your body hair to fall out.) The serious cardiovascular side effects of the earliest drugs to treat metastatic prostate cancer, for example, estrogens such as diethylstilbestrol (DES), have been eliminated by replacement with newer drugs. However, some of these newer drugs can cause gastrointestinal side effects, diarrhea being the most common. These symptoms can be overcome with over-the-counter remedies in most cases.

The biggest drawback to hormone therapy is that the prostate cancer cells gradually become immune to the treatment, or hormone resistant.

Why Cells Become Immune to Treatment

Your brain is the body's control center and the hypothalamus, at the base of the brain, secretes LHRH–luteinizing hormone-releasing hormone. LHRH flows to the nearby pituitary gland and prompts it to secrete luteinizing hormone–LH–which then circulates to your testicles and triggers the production of testosterone. Most testosterone is produced by the testicles and is the primary androgen. However, the pituitary gland not only secretes LH, it also releases ACTH–adrenocorticotropic hormone–which causes the adrenals to produce some of the body's androgens, about 5 to 10 percent of the total.

When androgens leave the testicles and adrenals and enter the prostate, they go through a transformation with the help of another enzyme, 5-alpha reductase. This enzyme converts testosterone to a more potent androgen called dihydrotestosterone–DHT.

When the brain gets the message that there is enough testosterone in the blood, it alerts the pituitary. This negative feedback mechanism decreases further release of LH from the pituitary, thereby controlling blood testosterone levels.

When this testosterone production system is shut down either by orchiectomy or drug manipulation, prostate tumors usually shrink, but after a while they start growing again. The hormone-dependent cells are very sensitive to testosterone, and without it they quickly shrink or degenerate. If all the prostate cells were this type, we would be able to cure prostate cancer with hormonal therapy.

But there are cancer cells that are androgen resistant or hormone independent. They are not affected at all by the presence or absence of androgens. These cells pose the biggest problem because they continue to grow and multiply no matter what hormonal manipulation is tried. They form clones of themselves and ultimately dominate the others. The cancer then becomes hormone refractory, or insensitive to hormone therapy. Many prostate cancers will become hormone refractory after 2 or 3 years of hormone treatment. When a man is diagnosed with hormone-refractory prostate cancer, it often indicates that he has metastatic disease and will show clinical signs of relapse after initial hormone therapy, with the PSA escalating rapidly over time.

Orchiectomy

Surgical removal of the testicles—the testosterone factory—stops production of 90 to 95 percent of testosterone. This surgery is called orchiectomy. Urologists do fewer orchiectomies now that drugs (medical or pharmacological treatment) have taken their place. Given a choice, the majority of men do not want to lose their testicles, even though the drug treatment takes more time and money.

Other than loss of the libido, there are no significant side effects to orchiectomy. It is an outpatient procedure that takes about 30 minutes with local or spinal anesthesia. An incision is made in the scrotum and the testicles are cut from the cords that connect them to the body. Blood vessels are cut and tied and the small incision in the scrotum is sewn back together. In the past, silicone prostheses were placed in the scrotum to fill the space of the lost testicles, but the potential harmful effects of silicone ended that practice.

Orchiectomy is sometimes followed up with the addition of antiandrogens such as flutamide (Eulexin) that block the androgen receptor so that the action of androgens from the adrenal gland will be blocked.

A 62-year-old man did not want to come to the office all the time for shots, so he opted for orchiectomy. His cancer had already spread to the lymph nodes and radical prostatectomy was not an option. He also had severe asthma and some hypertension, which could have put him at additional risk during surgery. Otherwise, he had a good life and made a living as an author. The orchiectomy was done 7 years ago and he still has no symptoms. However, his PSA is now 20 and he is seeing an oncologist to initiate adjuvant therapy.

Synthetic Hormones

A variety of drugs are used by themselves or in combination. Some are used intermittently for long or short periods of time. As with all treatment for prostate cancer, hormonal treatment is loaded with controversy. It can also be extremely expensive. This list identifies some of the commonly used drugs:

Estrogen
Diethylstilbestrol (DES)

LHRH Agonists/Antagonists
Leuprolide (Lupron)
Goserelin (Zoladex)

Antiandrogens
Flutamide (Eulexin)
Bicalutamide (Casodex)
Nilutamide (Nilandron)

Estrogen

In the 1960s, the Veterans Administration began treating prostate cancer patients with a synthetic form of estrogen, a female hormone, to avoid surgical removal of the testicles. Diethylstilbestrol (DES) blocks the production of testosterone from the testicles by preventing the release of LH from the pituitary gland.

Within 14 days of beginning treatment with DES, testosterone levels drop. It is taken in pill form, usually once a day. However, it can cause nausea, vomiting, breast enlargement and tenderness, and a decrease in libido.

The worst side effect, however, is the cardiovascular complications. DES can cause serious heart or blood vessel problems in men such as stroke, blood clots, pulmonary embolism, and swelling in the legs. Research found that lower doses eased these effects but were not effective as therapy against prostate cancer.

The use of DES has been limited in recent years because of the cardiovascular side effects, and also because there are better drugs now. However, DES is still widely used in other countries, including England, to treat prostate cancer, primarily because it is less expensive than the newer drugs. (DES achieved notoriety in the 1960s when it was prescribed as a fertility drug to women who had difficulty getting pregnant. It caused many birth defects and a long-lasting class-action suit by the daughters of DES mothers ended in the 1990s.)

LHRH Agonists-Antagonists

In the 1980s, other drugs were developed to do what DES did but without the cardiovascular side effects. Lupron (leuprolide) and Zoladex are LHRH agonists-antagonists that do not produce heart symptoms, although they can cause hot flashes, enlarged breasts, and loss of libido.

An LHRH agonist-antagonist is a synthetic drug designed to act like the real hormone and counteract the hormone at the same time. How does it do both? Lupron causes LH to increase to such a degree that in time it overwhelms the capacity of the pituitary gland to release LH. Then LH shuts down. If Lupron is taken without a prior course of antiandrogens, this initial flareup can make pain worse if there is any bone metastasis. It is like giving a shot of testosterone in the spine. The surge of hormone causes the cancer to press on the nerves and could cause paralysis.

LHRH agonists-antagonists are dispensed by a monthly injection in the doctor's office at a cost of more than $400 per shot plus the cost of visiting the doctor. Newer drugs with longer half-lives (they remain active longer) have been recently developed and these require only quarterly injections.

In a small number of patients, LHRH agonists-antagonists may cause testosterone to rise initially due to an increase in LH before it begins to fall. This surge, or flare response, lasts for a week or two.

Antiandrogens

Antiandrogens do not stop the production of androgens, but they stop their action by blocking the hormone receptor. Think of a medieval knight with a shield to block the blows of swords and arrows. This shield keeps the androgens away from the cancer cells.

Antiandrogens came into use in 1989, with Eulexin being the first. More recently, Nilandron and Casodex have come into use after years of clinical studies. The newer drugs with a longer half-life can be taken in pill form once a day. Eulexin requires a dose of two pills three times a day.

Not all patients have the same side effects to the same degree, but Eulexin causes diarrhea in about 20 percent of men. This side effect is more severe for men who are lactose intolerant; for example, many Asians have a common genetic intolerance for milk products. Diarrhea can often be managed with over-the-counter remedies and lots of fluids. Changes in diet can also help, such as cutting back on dairy products, eating smaller but more frequent meals, and consuming more carbohydrates such as bananas, rice, applesauce, or toast.

Alcohol consumption is not compatible with Nilandron. Casodex appears to be easier to tolerate than Nilandron or Eulexin, but there is more potential for cardiovascular toxicity. Ask your urologist about the latest hormonal drugs. By the time you read this book, there may be new ones available.

Maximal Androgen Blockade (MAB)

To counteract the initial flare of testosterone, antiandrogen drugs such as Eulexin were developed. These were given for 2 weeks before the LHRH agonists-antagonists to prevent the flare response. This combination is used in various ways for maximal hormonal deprivation. Many oncologists advocate continued use of both an antiandrogen and an LHRH agonist-antagonist.

Using a combination of surgical or medical castration with an antiandrogen is called complete hormonal therapy, or MAB. This treatment virtually shuts off the body's supply of hormones and slows the growth of cancer. A National Cancer Institute clinical trial showed that men who took both an LHRH agonist-antagonist and antiandrogens lived an average of 6 months longer than men who received only the agonist.

This treatment is for patients with early advanced disease, when the cancer is just beginning to spread to the bones and lymph nodes. If treatment starts at the time of bone metastasis, then 10 percent of the men can expect to live at least 10 years, 31 percent for 5 years, and 50 percent for 3 years. All men are different, however, and many live much longer than expected.

The strategy of intermittent hormonal therapy is to outsmart the body's production of hormones and the cancer cells' ability to resist hormonal manipulation. We know the cells become resistant in time, so the idea is to stop the treatment before that happens and give the cells a chance to rest, while monitoring the PSA levels, before starting the drugs again. The goal is to drive down the PSA and keep it there. Nobody knows for sure when is the best time to reinstitute therapy.

It is hoped that this start-and-stop strategy will keep the cancer in limbo. There is concern that survival could, in fact, be shortened by the intermittent withdrawal of androgens. Let's say an androgen-dependent cancer cell is treated with an LHRH agonist and an antiandrogen such as Eulexin to achieve perfect control. The PSA is close to zero. In this case, stopping therapy could refuel the disease because testosterone levels could gradually increase.

The advent of the PSA blood test for tracking prostate cancer made intermittent therapy more viable. In the late 1990s, there have been clinical studies all over the United States and a great deal of hope and excitement that this therapy may be the future of prostate cancer treatment.

Other Strategies

Hormones are sometimes used in combination with other treatment. Sometimes it may be effective to shrink, or downstage, a prostate tumor before radiation, with 2 or 3 months of hormonal therapy. Although this neoadjuvant treatment may not be as effective with surgery, the stakes are different with radiation. The hormonal therapy may make the target smaller and there will be less radiation scatter affecting the bowel and bladder. LHRH agonists-antagonists such as Lupron or Zoladex are usually used in this therapy, but some physicians may use both the agonists-antagonists in combination with an antiandrogen.

Managing Hormone-Refractory Cancer

Research on prostate cancer is in high gear, and among the medical community there is a feeling of hope that in the next few years we will be able to cure and possibly prevent this enigmatic disease. But even without a cure we are improving treatment techniques every day.

It is a difficult task for a man and his doctor to treat prostate cancer that has metastasized and is resisting treatment. Both must decide when to go ahead with treatment—or stop. It is never good to give up hope. If we look back at the progress we have made in medical treatment in the 1990s, there is reason to believe we can make as much or more progress in the near future.

Despite the high response rate and potential survival benefit of primary hormonal therapy for patients with metastatic cancer, the disease will eventually progress in virtually all men. Managing this stage of the disease is difficult and men with advanced disease should also consult with a medical oncologist for chemotherapy treatment to slow the progress of the disease or relieve discomfort.

Reducing Circulating Androgens

For most men there are two hormonal maneuvers to be considered before moving on to an oncologist. One is maintaining primary suppression of androgens produced by the testicles and the second is the withdrawal of antiandrogens in men who have been treated with maximal androgen blockade. There is evidence that a significant drop in PSA levels will occur in up to half the patients when Eulexin is withdrawn. The mechanism of this response remains unclear, although there is some suggestion that the drug exerts a stimulatory effect through a mutated androgen receptor.

The response rates for secondary hormonal therapies have been studied for more than 50 years, are highly variable, and should be interpreted with some caution. More recently, PSA levels have been shown to be valid indicators of response. Therefore, after secondary hormonal manipulation, PSA should be used to follow up the response to therapy.

Secondary Orchiectomy

If production of androgens was suppressed with drugs but is no longer working, orchiectomy should be considered. Secondary orchiectomy used in men with hormone-refractory prostate cancer after initial hormonal therapy shows a response rate of from 5 to 7 percent.

Corticosteroids

Corticosteroids are hormones that suppress the pituitary gland's production of adrenocorticotropic hormone (ACTH), which results in decreased production of androgens by the adrenal glands. Studies have shown improvement in hormone-refractory prostate cancer with this drug. In one study evaluating pain and quality of life, 38 percent of men improved after 1 month of treatment with oral prednisone. This reduction of symptoms is associated with the suppression of adrenal androgens. Response rates range from 20 to 80 percent, with the best estimate between 20 and 30 percent. This rate is determined by the reduction of bone pain, improvement in the quality of life, and feelings of wellness.

Ketoconazole

Ketoconazole is an antifungal agent shown to inhibit testicular and adrenal production of androgens. It is also believed to have a direct toxic effect on prostate cancer cells. Studies have shown a clinical response rate between 20 and 30 percent. However, ketoconazole produces side effects such as nausea, vomiting, skin rash, and breast enlargement.

Aminoglutethimide

Like ketoconazole, aminoglutethimide suppresses adrenal androgen production. This drug is usually administered with steroids and the response rate is from 20 to 40 percent. Side effects include lethargy, nausea, vomiting, skin rash, and breast enlargement.

Responses to secondary hormonal therapy are primarily subjective in nature and there is no evidence that any of these therapies increase survival or have consistent palliative effects. Men with hormone-refractory cancer should be enrolled in clinical trials designed to develop new therapies. (See Appendix 8 for a summary of clinical trials.) For those who are ineligible or unwilling to consider a trial, a second hormonal intervention is not unreasonable. The choice of therapy depends on many factors including other illnesses, prior hormonal therapy, and performance status.

A 58-year-old business manager discovered prostate cancer 4 years ago when it had already metastasized to his bones. Although he had a small tumor and a moderate Gleason score, his PSA was 25. This man had a history of hypertension but no family history of prostate cancer.

He agreed to Lupron and Eulexin therapy for 18 months and his PSA dropped to 0.5. He joined a support group and spent time on the Internet communicating with others and learning all he could about prostate cancer. While on the hormonal therapy he developed painful swelling of the breasts and he began to feel very depressed about the medications' effect on his body image. His earlier motivation to live his life to the fullest began to diminish. After 18 months of maximum androgen blockage, his PSA began to rise, first to 2.3, then to 4.9 in 3 months. A CAT scan revealed the cancer had spread to his lymph nodes, but still he had no real symptoms, except for slight urgency with urination. When the Eulexin was withdrawn, his PSA went down again. He has had a difficult struggle, but has not given up hope. Had he never discovered the cancer, and had no treatment, he would have died from the disease years ago.

The Cost of Treatment

Hormonal therapy is expensive. Monthly shots at the urologist's office cost almost $400 per injection plus the cost of the office visit. If you also require treatment with an antiandrogen, add another $250 a month for pills. Additionally, there may be expenses for medications to reverse the side effects.

Hormonal therapy is covered by most health insurance. HMOs sometimes provide the drugs directly to your doctor, which lowers the cost. If you are uninsured or if your medical insurance does not cover this expense, there are ways to get financial aid. Most of the drug companies have some assistance programs for uninsured or indigent patients. Ask your urologist about programs that may help. Also ask the American Cancer Society as well as Cancer Care. Appendix 4 lists resources for financial aid for treatment.

PART FIVE

Making the Decision

14

Choosing Physicians and a Treatment Center

More than one physician may be involved in your treatment for prostate cancer: a urologist, possibly a radiation oncologist, and a pathologist who plays a critical role behind the scenes. These physicians, plus a roster of technicians, nurses, and other health care professionals, all lend their expertise and opinions along the way. Look for the best-quality health care you can find from your physicians and treatment center.

Finding a Urologist

A urologist specializes in diseases of the reproductive and urinary tract in men, women, and children. Although urology is a subspecialty of surgery, urologists also specialize in other areas. They have training in pediatric urology, urologic oncology, male infertility, erectile dysfunction, and voiding disorders. Because a urologist is also a surgeon and because there is so much controversy and differing opinions about treating prostate cancer, it is important to get a second opinion and sometimes even a third opinion.

Be sure you find a urologist with extensive experience in treating prostate cancer. Most of your care will be provided by this physician, so be sure you are satisfied with his or her skills and approach to treatment. The urologist will not only do prostate surgery or treat you with hormonal therapy, but will perform or supervise all of your screenings for prostate cancer.

If you have no primary care physician or urologist, call a health network referral service or medical center in your area and ask for a urologist with experience in treating prostate cancer. When you call a doctor for the first time, ask for his or her credentials if you cannot find them out on your own. Be sure that all of your treatment team members—urologist, radiation oncologist, pathologist—are board certified.

In order to be certified by the American Board of Urology (ABU), a urologist must have completed an accredited residency program for a minimum of 5 years. Training includes surgery, clinical urology, and other relevant disciplines. Before certification, the physician must pass a regimen of written and oral examinations.

A doctor's background can be checked by calling the county medical society or the state medical board, or by consulting the medical directory at the reference desk of your public library. In some states it is now legal to check with the state board of medical examiners for a physician's profile and learn of any malpractice suits, disciplinary actions, and criminal history. You can also call the American Board of Medical Specialty in Chicago at 1-800-776-2378 to check on certification.

If you have confidence in your urologist, you may also feel confident about other specialists he or she recommends for treatment. However, before you meet these new doctors, ask some questions about the experience, reputation, and personality of the new physicians. If you are warned that a particular radiotherapist seems aloof or patronizing but has a top-notch reputation among his or her peers, you will not be expecting warmth and compassion when you interview this doctor. On the other hand, if you really dislike a doctor, you will not trust him or her and you should keep looking. You need to communicate openly with your physician, so do not compromise on the doctor's active participation in listening to you and helping you understand what your treatment involves.

When you meet a doctor for the first time, bring your wife or partner, as well as your medical records and family health history. There are many things to talk about: your laboratory results, your health history, the side effects of your treatment, your follow-up care. There are big "ifs" lurking in your mind, and you have a right to expect your doctor to help you answer them. What you want most when you are faced with a serious illness and treatment is help. You want someone to give you only the best information and advice.

Before you go to a first meeting with a new doctor, ask how much time you will be given for this meeting. In many health care plans, doctors limit the time they can spend with each patient, some granting less than

15 minutes. Also ask if you can begin your interview before the doctor visits you in the examination room. This way, you get a chance to know the doctor and ask some questions when you are not sitting naked or partially disrobed in the examination room, feeling more vulnerable. When you are dressed it is easier to question the doctor further or disagree with something.

Let doctors know you want the truth, not reassurance, no matter how comforting that may seem. Taking charge of your cancer treatment is the only way you can feel confident that you are doing all the right things to treat it. Don't lose track of the goal of treatment, which is to treat your prostate cancer and recover.

Your choice of urologic surgeon is directly related to your choice of treatment center. If you know where you want to receive your treatment, there may be several equally qualified urologists from which to choose. You may have less choice if you know which physician you want and he or she is only affiliated with one or two medical centers.

Prostate surgery is complex and requires a great deal of follow-up care. It also has considerable impact on your life, from the time needed for recovery, to possibly adapting to a new way of experiencing sex. Surgical skill is an extremely important factor in the outcome of prostate surgery. Complication rates vary considerably, so always find a urologist who specializes in prostate surgery and who has been doing it for many years, preferably in a major teaching hospital where there is access to the latest technology and equipment if complications arise.

Comprehensive Cancer Treatment Centers

Some community hospitals provide excellent health care, but they are often not equipped to provide the best available treatment for cancer. Depending on where you live, you may need to seek the best treatment in another town or city. You are most likely to get state-of-the-art prostate cancer treatment at a comprehensive cancer center at a teaching hospital.

A comprehensive cancer center is usually but not always part of a university hospital medical center. A teaching hospital will be able to offer a multidisciplinary treatment team approach to care, which means you could find a urologist, radiation oncologist, as well as other providers who work together to coordinate patient care.

At many teaching hospitals a "tumor board" meets regularly to discuss a multidisciplinary approach to cancer care. Such a board may include urologists, clinical oncologists, radiation oncologists, oncology nurses, and hospital social workers who share information. Your case is very likely to be discussed during these conferences and this information sharing can enhance the quality of your care. Academic physicians as well as the clinical physicians and other staff involved in your care all have input. This process is not like receiving health care by committee, however. Your personal physician is still in charge of your care.

In large cities where you have more choices you may be able to choose from several well-known teaching hospitals. If you must choose between two hospitals, a good rule of thumb is to ask about residency training programs. If the hospital has an approved residency training program in urology and radiation oncology, it means there are an adequate number of properly trained faculty members to supervise treatment. Some of the services available at a comprehensive cancer center include:

Diagnostic imaging center approved by the American College of Radiology

Pathology laboratory services

Pharmacy dedicated to cancer patients

Radiation treatment center

Psychiatric oncology: specialists to help with emotional concerns about treatment

Cancer hotline for the latest information

Nutritional service for treatment and prevention of cancer

Social work program to help you and your family cope with fears and anxieties and connect you with support groups or counseling

Support Services at Treatment Centers

Medical centers provide much more self-help or patient education today than they did in the past. Clinical nurse specialists often work exclusively with cancer patients and they are very helpful during surgery recovery in the hospital. They can teach you how to care for yourself when you get home and can recommend support groups and anything else you need, such as written materials and videos to help you understand and cope with treatment and side effects. Hospital social workers can assist you in finding a support group or other programs to help you and your family make the adjustment to dealing with prostate cancer. Most hospitals have a patient service representative. This person—or department if it is a large medical center—is the liaison between you and the hospital, helping with any problem or question you may have. Seek out this person with questions about the hospital's charges for your care or any procedures or people involved in your care in the hospital.

There is also a patient's bill of rights published by the American Hospital Association in 1973. All accredited hospitals must accede to this bill, which covers all patient concerns from quality of care to securing information and recognizing your right to privacy.

In addition to the right to quality care regardless of source of payment, age, religion, or ethnic origin, the patient's bill of rights outlines what you have a right to expect. For example, you have the right to decline treatment and leave the hospital against medical advice. If you want to go to another hospital, you have the right to expect the hospital to make that transfer possible. No one outside the treatment team and hospital has a right to see your medical records unless you say so. You have the right to know the name of all physicians involved in your care as well as other staff members. You have a right to information about your planned course of treatment, the probable length of hospital stay, and your prognosis for the future. You have the right to participate in decisions that affect your care. In addition, most states have laws concerning rights of medical patients. Find out from your patient services department or from the department of health in your state. Some hospitals post these rights in their lobby.

Psychiatric Oncology

Many cancer centers have specialists in psychiatric oncology, a program designed to help cancer patients cope with their disease and their treatment. There are group counseling programs as well as one-on-one programs. Hospital social workers can usually refer you to counselors.

Some medical centers also offer a variety of programs to help reduce the stress and pain involved in treatment. These include biofeedback, relaxation techniques, hypnosis, and acupuncture. See the next chapter for more information.

Many resources are available to help you through the process of treating prostate cancer, so take advantage of everything. There is more information in the next chapter of this book.

Paying for Treatment

Before you hand over your health insurance card, ask what your treatment will cost. A hospital billing clerk may be surprised by this request because so few patients ask. It may be up to you, in fact, to call your insurance company to inform them about any procedure you have. Some insurance companies will not cover you unless you notify them 24 hours in advance. The health care rules change daily and there are so many coverage plans that it is difficult to be sure what is covered, for how long, and by whom it must be referred.

Make sure you understand what and how much you are paying for. If you are responsible for partial payment—say a 20 percent copayment—according to your insurance coverage, it could add up to a substantial amount. And if you choose a doctor outside your health plan, it could become an overwhelming financial burden. Some hospitals may request a copayment from you up front, or if you have a deductible that has not been met, they may ask for that amount.

In addition to the surgeon's fee, there are hospital charges. You will be billed for use of the operating room, anesthesia, medications, the recovery room, your own room, and an assortment of miscellaneous charges. Ask the hospital for a list of standard charges for all procedures you have so that you are not surprised later. You may be asked to sign a consent form, agreeing to pay charges not covered by insurance. If you are too preoccupied to worry about this matter, have your partner or someone from your family oversee this process.

If You Belong to an HMO

The majority of the medically insured population is now enrolled in a managed care insurance program, mostly through their place of employment. It is important that you understand how HMOs affect your treatment options. Most people know very little about their health insurance plans other than the amount of their copayment. Problems relating to confusion about what the plans cover is becoming the norm.

HMOs generally require you to be treated only through referrals from your primary care physician, which can limit your choice of specialists and treatment options for prostate cancer. You may be restricted only to the physicians listed in your HMO directory—that is, you cannot visit a radiation oncologist or surgeon unless that physician is in the same plan and is referred by your primary care physician. If you consult and use a specialist outside the HMO network, your insurance company may not want to pay. (Keep in mind that you may be able to negotiate payment in certain cases and that many physicians will help you get the coverage you need.) Sometimes HMO restrictions also mean you can seek treatment only in your own neighborhood, city, or state. You may prefer to go to a city where there is a state-of-the-art cancer treatment center.

Be sure you understand which physicians must be referred by your primary care physician. Your state laws may be changing this situation. In some states it is now illegal to restrict choice of specialist and you can go to anyone you want. If you choose to seek a urologist with a good reputation for treating prostate cancer despite referral limitations, you may be covered. Always check on the details of your coverage.

Understand what your plan covers, but do not accept inferior treatment because of your HMO limitations. Call your insurance company, your physicians, and the hospital patient services department to find alternatives. Almost everything is negotiable if you persist, but it takes energy. Here again, you may want help from your family or friends.

There is a newly emerging occupation of health care consultant prompted by the proliferation of health care plans. Just as we need tax consultants because the system is complicated, we now need someone to help us through the maze of health care regulations. For a fee these consultants offer to take care of all of your insurance problems, from erroneous billing, to rejected claims, to fighting for the doctor or treatment you want. For information about these consultants, check with your lawyer, accountant, or corporate benefits department. Also look in your Yellow Pages under "Medical Claims Processing Services," or "Insurance Claims Processing Services."

Medicare and Medicaid

If you qualify for Medicaid or Medicare, then in theory you should have all costs covered. Medicaid coverage varies from state to state, however, and there are some private or community hospitals that will not accept Medicaid, so patients are sent to municipal or county facilities, which may not be the best source for care.

Call your local Department of Social Services to check on your eligibility for Medicaid or Medicare. If you are over 65, call the Agency for the Aging in your community.

There is more information on health insurance in Appendix 5.

15

Nonmedical Aids to Treatment

Even though early prostate cancer can be cured and impotence can be overcome, most men are devastated by the threat prostate cancer poses not only to their lives but to their identity as men. Many believe it would be easier to cope with lung cancer or a heart attack. Prostate cancer means castration! or wetting your pants! And the number of treatment options and controversy surrounding them add to the anxiety.

The diagnosis and treatment of prostate cancer, both short term and long term, can compromise your self-esteem, disrupt your family life, interfere with your job, and send your anxiety level through the roof. You may focus on the negative—the fact that prostate cancer is not curable, that you might die, that you will never have an erection again, that you are no longer a man, that you will have to wear diapers!

How you cope with this new stress has much to do with how you handle any stressful situation in your life. It is different for everybody, but the stress and anxiety should be handled. Otherwise, the process of getting treated and recovering will not be nearly as comfortable—or successful. You need help overcoming the stress and turmoil so that you can concentrate on getting better, overcoming the obstacles of temporary incontinence, and learning new ways to achieve an erection. As you learn more and become familiar with the treatment routine, your anxiety will diminish. You may also find renewed intimacy and affection with your spouse or partner. You will certainly learn a great deal about your body and medical care, and meet new people along the way.

Any serious illness concerns both you and your spouse or partner, but prostate cancer, with its possible sexual adjustments, puts a stronger emphasis on the need for honest communication with the most intimate person in your life. It is extremely important not to go through this alone. Even if you are single and live alone, there are people all around—if you look for them—who can help you.

Support from Family and Friends

If you already have a warm and loving circle of family and friends, you are in luck. But face it, your cancer can cause them stress, too, and put up road blocks in communication. Sometimes people will not know what to say or do, and often they do and say nothing for fear of making you feel worse. It's always a good idea to be precise and specific. Explain to your family exactly what your surgery and recuperation mean. Share with them what you have learned.

Try to communicate your feelings and needs. If you want their help or moral support, ask for it. Often we expect those we love to read our minds and provide all kinds of comfort and support. But it is better if we ask. As a rule, men do not generally pour out their hearts as easily as women. They seem to have a more difficult time asking for help. If you live alone, maybe you want some company or a ride to your radiation treatments. Sometimes you may just want someone to hang out with you. If you do not have people to ask, talk with your physician or treatment team. They will be able to connect you with a network of people available to help you recover from prostate cancer.

In the Workplace

How much you share with people you work with depends on them and on you, as well as on the nature of your work. If you are in a high-stress job, such as a Wall Street securities analyst or a trial attorney, where your image has a lot to do with your performance, then you may not want to talk with any of your co-workers about your illness and treatment. If you work in the helping professions, it might be easier for you to share some of your feelings with people around you.

You may be undergoing radiation therapy or hormonal therapy while you are working. You may be wearing an absorbent pad or incontinence pants that make you feel awkward. If there are people with whom you can share confidences on the job, then let them know what you are going through. One of the best things to do is tell your co-workers what is going on before your treatment and keep in touch with them right after your surgery or during radiation therapy. Let them know that what you are doing is only temporary, like being treated for any other disease, that you are looking forward to coming back to work, and that you appreciate their concern. Educate them about prostate cancer and your treatment so that they will understand what you are dealing with—and what you are not dealing with. If you must come in late or leave early, or if you use your lunch hour for radiation treatments, say you are getting treatment but you expect to be fine.

You may be in a large organization where there are already many other cancer survivors. In that case, you may want to seek out others, perhaps even form a workplace support group. This can be a way to find mutual emotional support and it may provide a forum for those co-workers who learn that they have cancer.

Support Groups

Even a loving family and friends are not always enough. You need to talk with other men who know what it's like to have prostate cancer. You may enjoy the camaraderie and you could also be a good role model for another person.

Cancer support groups can offer one of the best ways to get yourself through a rough time. They help you feel less anxious, less depressed, less afraid, and thus you may experience less pain. It's a place where you can feel safe and secure, where everybody understands what you are going through. You don't have to be stoic and hide your fears behind macho posturing. There is no substitute for the emotional bond that develops among people in a dynamic cancer support group.

You can find practical help about how other men cope with their jobs, families, or friends who don't know what to say or do. You can find out how other men adapted and enhanced their sexuality. Your partner or spouse can find comfort in this group, too, by learning about other partners in the same situation.

On the negative side, newly diagnosed men may find some support groups too intense. For example, a group in New York City is full of high-powered men who take a very aggressive stance about everything in their lives. This kind of intensity may depress you if you have been cured with early-stage cancer. But don't give up until you have the opportunity to talk with some of the other men in the group. Ask about what they like and dislike about the group.

Most cancer centers have or know of a chapter of Us Too, International, for men with prostate cancer. This organization was started in 1990 by a group of men who needed to understand treatment options for prostate cancer. Now, with more than 60,000 members in 400 chapters all over the world, Us Too has become not only a support group but an advocacy group to raise awareness about the needs of men with prostate cancer. Meetings are open to members and their families, and very often specialists in the care and treatment of prostate cancer come to meetings to provide information about surgery, radiation, nutrition, and other aspects of care. If there are no Us Too chapters in your area, think about starting one. Us Too relies on volunteers to set up new chapters. This takes a lot of work but may be rewarding.

Call your local American Cancer Society chapter for information about the *Man to Man* program, which sponsors support groups and also has a one-on-one visitation program. This program arranges for a specially trained prostate cancer survivor to come and talk with you personally about the experience of prostate cancer. It is not a medical program but an opportunity to talk with another man who has gone through what you are going through. This approach may be more appealing to you if you are not inclined to talk about yourself in a group.

To find a support group near you, ask at your hospital social work department or call the Cancer Information Center at the National Cancer Institute for the booklet *Taking Time: Support for People with Cancer and the People Who Care About Them.*

Check Appendix 1 for phone numbers and Internet addresses.

Private Counseling

If you are not willing to talk about your feelings in a support group or to another survivor, you may feel more comfortable talking privately with a psychologist or psychiatrist for some short-term counseling while you are going through your treatment. Many comprehensive cancer treatment centers now routinely offer this service. There is a newly developing therapeutic specialty called psychiatric oncology.

Psychiatric oncology is the result of increasing recognition by the health care establishment that cancer patients have unique emotional needs as well as potential psychological problems to address. The illness and the treatment interact with other emotional needs, cultural background, work, marriage, and family life.

More often than not, short-term counseling—once or twice a week—is all that is needed to get you through the therapeutic process. Counseling can be one-on-one with your therapist or it can include your spouse, partner, or family member. Your local hospital oncology or psychiatry department, social worker, or patient services representative should be able to help you locate a therapist. Otherwise, call the American Medical Association, the American Psychiatric Association, or the American Psychological Association.

Reducing the Stress of Living with Cancer

Anyone who has had cancer—any kind of cancer—generally comes away from the experience with a new perspective on life. Once cancer has been in your body, you always feel vulnerable, whether you are cured or given only 2 years to live. Nobody can ever be sure that a cancer cell has not escaped detection and won't turn up later. What cancer survivors share is the knowledge of how fragile life really is and that the purpose of life is to live it to the fullest every day.

The medical establishment has begun to recognize alternative treatments that can help patients reduce anxiety so that they can live full lives. These treatments have been used to reduce stress-induced heart attack and stroke, as well as cancer pain. Some cancer centers may offer behavioral therapy such as visualization, biofeedback, and relaxation techniques that help you cope and feel in control of your treatment and recovery. There are many effective techniques, from acupuncture to hypnosis to Zen meditation, but here are some that are recognized by health professionals as the most effective.

• **Biofeedback.** This technique teaches you to monitor your own muscle tension and then intervene to relax that tension and reduce anxiety. Electrodes attached to your skin monitor subtle changes in temperature, muscle, perspiration, blood pressure, and heart rate and rhythm. By observing what your muscles are doing—signals from the electrodes form graphs on a video screen—you can learn to intervene and change them. Biofeedback can also help you to reduce the level of pain you are feeling. Most large hospital psychiatry departments and an increasing number of cancer centers have a biofeedback therapist on staff. Medical insurance often covers this therapy. Biofeedback is also used to help patients regain continence after prostate surgery.

• **Visualization.** This technique is also known as guided imagery. With instruction and training, some patients can achieve a relaxed state by imagining they are in a more pleasant situation, such as lying on a beach or floating in an expanse of calm water. Cancer patients are often helped to imagine their cancer cells being knocked out by their radiation or hormonal medications. By putting themselves into this kind of state before or during their treatments, patients can often make the experience more pleasant and feel more positive that their treatment is succeeding. Men can also try to visualize themselves free of pain or stress, which can be an effective way to meet a challenge such as cancer treatment.

• **Meditation.** For centuries, people have been practicing meditation to achieve a higher level of consciousness and thus rid their psyches of stress and achieve a level of calm acceptance (nirvana). More and more health professionals recommend it as a way to manage stress and pain. There are no hard-and-fast rules on how to meditate. Not everyone needs to sit on the floor for hours in the lotus position, which may be difficult to achieve if you are recovering from surgery. The most important aspect is to close your eyes, breathe in and out slowly, and concentrate on each breath as you let all your thoughts fall away. There are many books and videos available to help you learn meditation techniques and how to achieve a relaxed and tranquil state of mind.

• **Eastern Techniques.** People from Asian cultures have a different perspective about illness and the body. The yin and yang philosophy, for example, is about harmony and balance, and their approach to bringing themselves back into balance involves a variety of methods. Chinese herbal medicine is more than 6,000 years old and still going strong. The Chinese use herbs as we use vitamins—to make up for a deficiency or give them strength. Tai chi is like a physical therapy for restoring balance to your body. Acupuncture is used for everything from quitting smoking to reducing chronic pain.

There is a great deal available today to aid you on your voyage through cancer treatment. Take advantage of everything to make your cancer treatment more positive and comfortable—and to help you live each day to the fullest.

16

Making Your Decision

Because there are so many variables, so many treatment options, and so much controversy surrounding prostate cancer, choosing the treatment that is best for you has been called the decision from hell. To add to your dilemma, there could be even more choices available by the time you read this book. As research studies and clinical trials reach their completion in the early 21st century, we may have more knowledge and insight into treatment.

Before we had transrectal sonograms and PSA tests, physicians could only discover prostate cancer when patients became symptomatic or when the DRE was abnormal, and by then the cancer was usually advanced and there were few treatment options. Now, with our sophisticated screening techniques and more awareness about early detection, we have created another dilemma. We can find microscopic disease, but we still do not know with certainty what it will do. How do we know who has the aggressive cancer that may progress rapidly and cause early death, or who has a cancer that will grow so slowly that he will die first from something else?

It is especially important with prostate cancer to learn all you can before you decide. Some men still accept whatever recommendations are handed to them by their doctors, but more and more men are now beginning to take responsibility and seek out information. They compare recommendations from doctors with what they learn from others who have had the disease and with what they turn up in their own research in libraries, on the Internet, and with the help of support groups.

Because there are often no symptoms with early prostate cancer, treating it aggressively with surgery or radiation is meant to prevent the cancer from spreading. However, because prostate cancer has a very slow doubling time in most cases, the cancer may take a decade or more to spread outside the prostate. Many men will likely die of other conditions such as heart disease before the prostate cancer ever catches up with them. For this reason, it is sometimes considered prudent to simply maintain surveillance of the condition through regular DRE and PSA testing. On the other hand, the opportunity for cure exists only while the cancer is contained within the prostate gland.

Many variables guide your treatment choice—volume of tumor, Gleason score, PSA level, your general health, and presence or absence of metastases. Some of these variables will become obvious after initial screening whereas others will not until after clinical biopsy or surgery. For example, you cannot know if cancer has invaded your lymph nodes until they are removed surgically and analyzed.

The Gleason score is important because we can assume that a high-grade cancer (Gleason 8, 9, 10) is more likely to progress and spread faster to other organs. On the other hand, a low-grade cancer (Gleason 2, 3, 4) may not move out of the prostate for many years.

The volume of the tumor is also a critical factor. Once a prostate carcinoma approaches 3 cubic centimeters it may break through the prostate capsule into the seminal vesicles and neurovascular bundle. However, a tumor generally has to be larger than 4 cubic centimeters before it metastasizes to distant locations. Most urologists believe there are essentially three yardsticks regarding treatment choice: age, stage of cancer, and whether or not you expect to live 10 or more years.

Your treatment choice will depend not only on the dynamics of your prostate cancer but on your age, your temperament, your general health, and where you live in relation to treatment centers. In these variables as well as in the clinical variables every man is unique.

All treatment choices will produce side effects, so it is important to weigh them carefully and imagine how they will affect your lifestyle. Even if you choose watchful waiting, you could have emotional side effects caused by worry, or you could miss out on a chance for surgery later if your health deteriorates. With surgery or radiation treatment you could be made temporarily or permanently incontinent or impotent. Can you live with that possibility? Some men don't care, but others would rather die than risk sexual dysfunction. With hormone treatment you may experience hot flashes, breast enlargement, and loss of libido. You need to figure out the trade-off with each type of treatment and how you would handle it.

Try not to get caught up in the emotional angst of wondering how you got prostate cancer—poor diet, living near a chemical dump, or your own failure to get early screening. Forget all that. You cannot change it now. And science does not know yet what causes prostate cancer. Now is the time to get all the information you can, make a decision you feel comfortable with, and focus on treating and recovering from the cancer. Once you have made your decision, you cannot look back. Doing so would only add a negative dimension to your ability to cope with prostate cancer.

Getting More Medical Opinions

It is quite likely that your urologist will recommend the best treatment, but don't be rushed. Now is the time to get all the information and support you need, as well as a second or third opinion. Be aware that doctors have biases. Because urologists are surgeons, they may believe more strongly in surgery as the best treatment. Radiation therapists naturally believe their treatment is best. A good doctor will encourage you to become well informed and even guide you in seeking other opinions before you make such an important decision.

You may get completely different opinions from two urologists, but each time you speak to someone new you will gain insight. After several conferences you will have a better understanding of your situation. It is the only way to become an informed patient. It is important that you believe you are really getting a second opinion and not just a carbon copy of the first one, which can happen when the first physician you talk with sends you to another colleague in the same practice or the same hospital—or even the same office. If your health insurer does not require a second opinion, you may have to pay for it yourself. But again, always negotiate for the best care possible.

When you visit doctors for additional opinions, bring your medical records. This is the most efficient way of communicating important medical information between physicians. Frequently, when you visit another doctor—even when you are referred by your urologist—your paperwork has not arrived. Ask for a copy of the report for each procedure you have: blood tests, pathology reports, and results of screenings you have had. These reports are part of your medical record and you are entitled to have copies. Many people mistakenly believe the records are the sole property of the doctor or hospital.

Because you are feeling vulnerable now, it may be hard to remain clear and objective. Bring along your wife or partner or a close friend for moral support. Write down your questions before you meet with each doctor so that you don't forget anything. Many people complain that doctors rush them. If you feel rushed when you visit a physician for a checkup or procedure, ask for another appointment so that you have additional time to ask questions and talk. It is quite common to think of questions after you get home and mull over everything the doctors have told you. Bring a notebook to keep track of the information you gather. There's nothing wrong with bringing a tape recorder to an interview if it helps you remember the answers given and allows you to compare opinions intelligently. This is a cram course and you are learning a whole new language.

Always ask the purpose of all treatment procedures. For example, treatment is usually aimed at curing the disease (curative), stemming its growth, or reducing symptoms (palliative). Understand how each procedure will affect your quality of life in the near and distant future.

If your cancer is advanced, ask your doctor to be honest with you. There used to be a belief among physicians that telling a seriously ill patient as little as possible and not confronting him with his own mortality was the most humane approach. Today we believe you have a right to know what to expect, what is the worst that can happen. You should receive comfort and candor from a doctor when you ask questions about how long you can expect to live or if you will get well again. Such questions should be answered in the most simple and direct way possible.

If the chance of your cancer recurring after treatment is 65 percent, for example, you should expect your doctor to explain what that means. Does it mean that in 5 years this percentage will diminish if your cancer has not recurred? Nobody can answer that question, which is what you should expect your physician to tell you. The percentages attached to stages are "guesstimates" based on what we know, which is incomplete at best. You might be among the 65 percent who have a recurrence in 5 years or among the 35 percent who never have a recurrence. Or the cancer could recur after a ten-year remission. Your immediate future can and should be charted, so it is wiser to take one step at a time.

Considering Your Other Medical Conditions

You may have reached an age where you have other medical conditions that can affect your treatment for prostate cancer. For example, if you have heart disease, surgery may be too risky for you. It is important to talk to your other doctors about your prostate treatment. Arrangements for your overall health care should be communicated among physicians. This is especially important if you have a preexisting heart, lung, or neurological condition in order to get fully evaluated prior to treatment. It will be up to you to get a dialog going among your doctors and have them coordinate your care.

If you are getting radiation therapy, you will need to know how much of your care will be transferred to your radiation therapist. Who should you call if you get a numbness or tingling in your groin or on your side— your radiation oncologist or your urologist, your primary care physician or your cardiologist? Is the numbness or tingling from the radiation or from hormonal drugs, or is it from your heart condition? One of the pitfalls of having so many physicians is never being quite sure who to call with a question. However, most patients tend to call whichever doctor returns phone calls efficiently.

Ask your doctors ahead of time if they will take your calls in the days during the process of treatment. It is a good idea to find doctors who are not only competent but who will respond to your needs quickly. If you cannot reach your urologist and you can reach your radiation oncologist, for example, then ask that physician to put you in the hands of someone who can help with your immediate problem.

Copies of your test reports will be needed by other doctors during treatment and follow-up care. It is your responsibility to follow up. Make sure your urologist gets a copy of the report from your radiation oncologist. Some doctors will make sure a report is forwarded the day it is requested. Others may not be as prompt. The easiest and least stressful method is for you to get copies of your reports from your doctors as they are generated and carry them with you.

Considering Your Emotional Response

Whatever your background, you need to consider many things in addition to the treatment itself: your ability to cope with stress, where you live in relation to treatment centers, and the feelings of your wife or partner. It's also helpful to look at the big picture, rather than just at the treatment. Think of the process—before treatment, during treatment and after treatment. Try to imagine and think through all the steps in the process and how you will feel. Know that anger, fear, anxiety, and depression are part of the process. Be honest about your emotions and ask yourself some questions.

- What makes you comfortable and uncomfortable?
- Can you express fear, rage, and anger?
- Can you talk about intimate concerns with your family, your physicians, your colleagues at work, or strangers?
- Are you aware of your own denial? (If you are postponing following up with treatment and making the decision because you are too busy at work, you are in denial.)
- How do you usually cope with crisis? What about stress? Do you suffer in silence or find help?
- How do you adapt to change?
- What is your social environment? Are there people around you or are you totally alone and isolated?
- Do you want to know everything about your disease, or not?
- How important is sex? Would you enjoy sex if you had to learn new ways to achieve an erection?

Sharing Decision Making with Your Family

Because prostate treatment can have a major impact on your lifestyle, it is important to get your intimate partner involved in the discussions with doctors and talk over issues between yourselves. Both of you must express your opinions and feelings about how the treatment you choose will affect your future. Treatment can have lasting effects on your sex life and both of you need to be informed before deciding what to do.

A 52-year-old teacher had no symptoms of prostate cancer until his family doctor discovered his elevated PSA. This man and his wife had grown children and were ready to enjoy doing things together. His physician suggested he bring his wife to all meetings so that they could both learn what treatment would mean. With his wife involved in the process, the teacher felt less alone, less in a vacuum. When two people hear the same thing, they can talk it over and see if they both come away with the same opinions or different ones.

The teacher went through more diagnostic tests, including a CAT scan and bone scan to make sure his cancer did not appear anywhere else in his body. His clinical biopsy showed a Gleason score of 6, meaning his cancer was moderately aggressive. The teacher and his wife decided on surgery. They both want him to live as long as possible. Neither one wanted to live wondering if the disease would progress and kill him.

The cooperation of your partner and family is essential to your recovery. If your activities must be restricted, for instance, tell them how this will affect your participation in family life and what you would like them to do for you. Just as successful treatment comes from a cohesive medical team, the same team effort will be needed from your family for your recovery.

Patients sometimes try to protect their families from the details, but this makes everyone more anxious. Your brothers, or sons, or even your father may be concerned about their own vulnerability for prostate cancer. Most people know very little about prostate cancer and it can be devastating news. They may think the worst—that they will lose you. If you are candid with your family and friends about how you feel and what you need from them, everyone will cope better. Explain what is going on so that they don't hear it from others who may be misinformed. Once people know you have prostate cancer, you will hear a hundred stories about anyone who ever had it and what happened to them. These stories may bear little relevance to your particular case and treatment options.

Proximity to Treatment Centers

In real estate, location is everything. In health care, it can also play a critical role. You may live in an area with only a small community hospital or you may live in a city with a larger hospital but without a comprehensive cancer treatment center. You can go to another city for surgery, but what about the 8 or 9 weeks of radiation? Even if you can relocate for daily treatment, can you take the time off from work?

Many men travel to other cities to get the best treatment. It is important that you feel confident that the treatment you get is the best there is. When you investigate cancer treatment centers, make sure they are experienced in dealing with patients with prostate cancer. Ask for data regarding treatment and the outcomes for various stages of the disease. Find out how many patients are comparable to you in age, family history, Gleason score, and TNM (tumor, nodes, metastasis) stage.

The Cost of Treatment

Surgical removal of the testicles—orchiectomy—is a one-time procedure that costs less than $1,000 and takes half an hour. But hormonal therapy with drugs can take years and cost almost $10,000 a year. Radiation therapy can cost tens of thousands of dollars. More specific information is given in the chapters of this book that describe particular treatments. Most insurance plans cover each type of prostate cancer treatment described here, but since all plans are different it is important that you find out in advance what your coverage includes so that you can get the best possible treatment. Sometimes the treatment itself may be covered, but the ancillary treatments, laboratory tests, or medications may not be covered. It is of critical importance to be familiar with your health coverage.

PART SIX

Recovery

17

Coping with Temporary Incontinence

Urinary incontinence following prostate cancer surgery or radiation treatment is rarely permanent. Most men have no problem after a few months, but about 30 percent have some degree of stress incontinence–leakage or dripping after an increase in intra-abdominal pressure when coughing or sneezing. With today's more advanced surgical techniques, permanent incontinence is extremely rare and occurs in about 3 percent of men.

The psychological problem is usually much worse than the physical problem. During the weeks or months of recovery you may need incontinence pants or pads to protect you from stress leaks and you may feel you are not in control of your own body, that you are like a baby wetting your pants. Perhaps you cannot play golf, or dance, or laugh out loud for fear of leaking or worse. And how do you enter a locker room or a public men's room without feeling mortified?

The encouraging news is that this incontinence is rarely permanent and there is a great deal that you can do to speed the process of complete recovery through special exercises and medications. There is no way to predict how long incontinence will last. Every man is different. It can take longer if you are older. Some men regain control in days whereas others need months. Nighttime continence always comes back first, because when you are lying down there is no pressure on the bladder or the sphincter and the pelvic floor. In time you may notice that you are sleeping longer through the night and your diaper is dry in the morning.

Before surgery you had two sphincter muscles that control the flow of urine. The internal sphincter, the one at the bladder neck, is the involuntary smooth muscle that is always at work without your conscious control. Because of the prostate's location at the base of the bladder and because the urethra passes through the prostate, the internal sphincter muscle is disrupted when the prostate is removed. The bladder neck itself, with its ring of muscles to control the flow of urine, may be completely removed in most cases. This sphincter is gone for good after radical prostatectomy. It is replaced by the anastomosis, the connection of the urethra to the bladder.

Without your internal sphincter muscle, continence depends entirely on the external sphincter. This skeletal muscle is located in the pelvic floor muscle, which is like a sling that supports the bladder and other organs. The external sphincter is the one that you are aware of, the one you tighten up when you want to stop the urinary stream, and the one you relax when you want urine to flow. This muscle may be weakened by surgery, but there are ways to retrain and strengthen it. When any part of this system fails, some type of incontinence can occur. There are several types of incontinence.

• **Stress incontinence** is the leakage of urine when you sneeze or cough. The increase in intra-abdominal pressure puts pressure on the bladder, causing the bladder neck to open. Stress incontinence can occur when you get up from a chair or lift a heavy object from the floor. Many people with stress incontinence avoid exercising because they are afraid to cause leaks.

• **Urge incontinence** is due to the involuntary contraction of the bladder muscle, which causes pressure in the bladder to increase, and this stimulates a reflex arc to the brain, telling you that you need to urgently go to the rest room or you will leak. Increased bladder pressure overcomes the sphincter's ability to maintain continence.

• **Overflow incontinence** occurs when the bladder has lost elasticity and cannot generate strong contractions to completely empty itself. Because it is never completely empty, additional urine production causes it to overflow, that is, to leak out.

• **Global incontinence** means there is no ability to control the flow of urine and the bladder constantly empties. This condition is extremely rare.

Functioning with a Catheter

A Foley catheter will extend from your penis for a few weeks after surgery so that urine will drain without putting any stress on your reconstructed lower urinary tract. A balloon attached to the other end of the catheter is inside your bladder to hold it in place. It will take up to 3 weeks for the anastomosis—the newly created connection of your urethra to your bladder neck—to heal.

The hospital staff will teach you how to manage the catheter so that the urine can drain into a bag without backing up. In fact, most hospitals cannot discharge you until they are confident you can operate the overnight bag and the leg bag.

While you sleep, the catheter drains into an overnight bag that is fastened to the lower part of the bed. When you get up or go out, you can connect the catheter to a leg bag that wraps around your thigh and will not show beneath your clothing. (Bring baggy trousers for the trip home to hide the bag. Put gauze pads in your underwear in case the catheter leaks.) It is strapped to your leg and is unobtrusive. However, this bag does not hold as much urine as an overnight bag, so you cannot allow it to get too full.

Don't worry if your catheter and leg bag get wet when you shower. Water will not hurt them. Be sure to keep the tip of your penis clean. Your penis and scrotum may be swollen for a while after surgery. When you are walking around, wear jockey shorts for support, and when you are resting, try to elevate your scrotum and penis by placing a rolled-up towel or pillow beneath them. It may be uncomfortable sleeping with a catheter, but you will adjust by finding the best position.

Urine will constantly drain during the first few weeks after surgery. It is not a start-and-stop action during this time. When you empty the receptacles, be aware of anything unusual and alert your physician if any of these problems occur:

- No urine has entered the bag for over 2 hours.
- The urine is dark red, cloudy, or foul smelling.
- Bladder spasms, which can be painful and cause squirts of urine

to leak around the catheter. (There is medication to relax the bladder.)

- Your catheter is clogged by clots or debris.

About 3 weeks after surgery, your physician will remove the catheter. Urination could be painful the first few times after the removal of the catheter.

Strengthening the External Sphincter

Kegel exercises are simple exercises that are extremely effective in strengthening your pelvic muscles and thus the external sphincter muscle and may accelerate the return of continence. The pelvic floor muscles act as a sling or a support for the bladder, keeping it elevated in place. When the muscles are weak, the organs drop down and become more difficult to control. Kegel exercises, which can be done anywhere and anytime, are the best way to restore your external sphincter muscle. Squeeze and release the muscles used to control urination and excretion. These squeezing maneuvers are the single most effective thing you can do to promote the return of continence.

How to Do Kegels

While urinating, try to stop the flow of urine to get some idea of how weak or strong your external sphincter muscle is. Then try to do Kegels every hour. Do them while sitting at your desk, reading, or watching TV.

While standing, squeeze and hold for 10 seconds. Breathe and count out loud. Relax for 10 seconds. Start and stop and gradually increase the number of squeezes. Repeat this exercise up to 15 times until you are too tired or unable to hold the squeeze for 10 seconds. They should be done 30 to 60 times a day for pelvic muscle rehabilitation. The more often you do these exercises, the sooner you will see results. They are especially effective if you do them when you are engaged in an activity that causes urine leakage, such as when you feel a cough or sneeze coming on, when you are about to get up from a chair, or when you lift something.

You might even keep a record or diary of how often you lose urine and what activities cause leakage so that you can be ready for it or practice a Kegel to try to prevent it. Such a record will also keep track of your progress. Make a chart for each day, for example, every 2-hour time frame. For each time period, record any incontinence episode—small or large—and the reason for it. For example, you sneezed or got up from a chair. Record the amount of liquid you drank and when or if you urinated. Keep track of the number of times you got up during the night to urinate. At the end of each day, record the total number of episodes.

Biofeedback

Biofeedback uses electrical and mechanical instruments to help patients retrain the pelvic floor muscle when it is weak or damaged. A tiny electric current is sent to the pelvic floor and bladder and prompts them to contract and get stronger. Biofeedback may be effective if you have trouble doing Kegel exercises. A therapist operates the equipment and teaches you how to monitor your progress.

While you are connected to the instrument and sensors, information is displayed on a video monitor about electrical impulses from your body. These sensors read electrical signals you create when you contract or relax your muscles. You see what is happening on the computer screen, which is how you learn to control the muscles. By watching how you learn to control your reaction, you are helping to reinforce appropriate responses. The therapist acts as a guide to help determine the correct behavior.

Diet Modification

All that you eat and drink creates urine. Naturally, the more you drink, the more you need to urinate. However, the logical step to reduce amounts of urine generated is not to stop drinking fluids. This can be dangerous. If you don't drink enough fluids, you can become dehydrated. It's important to maintain a balance and to know which foods and beverages create more urine and which ones do not.

Carbonated drinks, citrus fruits and juices, spicy foods, caffeine, and alcohol can irritate your bladder and increase the need to urinate. Some medications and drugs can have the same effect, for example, high-blood-pressure pills, sleeping pills, tranquilizers, antidepressants, sedatives, diuretics, antihistamines, decongestants, cold remedies, and some painkillers.

Using Protective Products

When the catheter is removed about 3 weeks after your surgery and until the urinary incontinence recedes you may need to use protection from involuntary leakage. Absorbent pads and external condoms are widely available. These products and devices should be considered temporary remedies. They should never be used in place of exercise and treatment, but they can make you feel more secure while you are going through the process. The cost of these items is covered by medical insurance, although you may have to file claims to get reimbursed.

• **Absorbent pads.** A variety of products can absorb urine whether it is a few drops or the entire contents of your bladder. There are pads that can be inserted into underpants, such as Depends Guards for Men. A bulkier and larger pad, with a waistband, is more like an undergarment. Then there are adult briefs, which are the bulkiest but offer total protection. They are fastened with self-adhesive tape. Bed pads are available in several sizes and degrees of absorbency.

• **External Condoms.** These are made of latex and are strapped on to collect urine, much like a catheter bag. When they fill up, they become heavy and can drop off if you do not tend to them right away.

Treating Severe Incontinence

In rare cases where incontinence is more severe, or if it is caused by other conditions combined with prostate cancer treatment, there are other options.

Collagen Implants

A synthetic polymer, very much like the body's natural collagen, can be used as a way to "bulk" the urethral tissue so that your muscles don't have to close such a wide gap to stop the flow of urine.

Although collagen implants do not work for everyone, and many physicians believe they are not a good solution to the problem, some physicians believe they can be effective for some men. The implanting is done in a hospital on an outpatient basis with local anesthesia.

A cystoscope is used for this procedure. This instrument is a fiberoptic tube with a telescope inserted into the penis that allows the physician to see inside the urethra. Then a needle is inserted through the cystoscope so that the synthetic collagen, Contigen, can be injected through the needle into the wall of the urethra near the bladder neck. The collagen builds up the wall of the urethra, closing the gap, which is called bulking the urethral tissue. The bulk creates a seal to stop leakage, but the tissue separates naturally when you need to urinate. A month later your doctor will examine you to see if you need more injections of Contigen.

Complications are rare, but there is the possibility that the implants could make the incontinence worse or close up the urethra too much so that urine cannot get out. Implants can sometimes cause pain and discomfort, an infection in the bladder or urethra, or an allergic reaction.

Artificial Sphincter

In rare cases of persistent or global incontinence, an artificial sphincter can be implanted after a radical prostatectomy. This silicone device has a cuff and a pump. The inflatable cuff wraps around the urethra to stop the flow of urine. The pump is implanted inside the scrotum. When you need to urinate, you squeeze the pump in the scrotum to deactivate the device and let the fluid out of the cuff. This deflates the cuff and allows urine to flow through the urethra. The cuff can then be inflated to restore urinary continence after voiding is completed.

Implanting an artificial sphincter is a very complicated and specialized surgery. Only urologists with special training and experience are qualified to do this procedure.

Complications can be with the mechanism itself, such as mechanical failure, or due to infection. The artificial sphincter is considered by most urologists to be a reasonable option for patients with incontinence and there is a high cure rate.

18

Restoring Potency After Prostate Cancer

The effects on a man's sex life of a radical prostatectomy or radiation therapy after prostate cancer can be profound, and very often he is not aware of many available options for restoring potency. Doctors often do not give their patients enough information about this subject and just as often men do not ask their doctors for help. It is vitally important for men to talk about their own experience and feelings, and to understand that if one method of restoring potency does not work for them, they can try another. Too often men become discouraged and fail to get adequate treatment.

Dr. J. François Eid, director of the Erectile Dysfunction Unit at the New York Hospital–Cornell Medical Center, has treated more than 8,000 men for erectile dysfunction and helped to organize the largest study ever done on restoring potency with penile injection therapy. He believes that men should be encouraged to resume sexual intimacy as soon as possible after treatment for prostate cancer. With the increase in early detection and radical prostatectomy in younger vigorous men, there is an even more urgent need to educate men about the options available to restore potency.

Radical prostatectomy and radiation therapy can injure the nerves and blood vessels critical to the erectile process, but in different ways. The neurovascular bundles located on the sides of the prostate may have been damaged during surgery in order to remove all the cancer. If both bundles are gone, the risk of impotence is higher. If only one is gone and you are young, you will probably remain potent. These are not the nerves that are involved in orgasm and sensation. While nerve-sparing prostate cancer surgery has improved the odds of retaining potency, most of the men who undergo radical prostatectomy have some degree of impotence for some time following surgery. As mentioned in the chapter on surgical treatment for prostate cancer, the younger the man, the more likely erectile function will return.

After radiation therapy, erectile dysfunction is gradual. This treatment accelerates atherosclerosis, which produces a reaction in the walls of the arteries. The arteries become thickened and the lumen (passageway) becomes obstructed. Radiation can leave blood vessels callused and scarred, and in this condition the vessels are unable to transport blood into the penis to achieve effective erectile function.

Some urologists believe it is better to let their patients recover from the surgery or radiation and wait and see what develops over the next several months or years. Others believe that waiting is not a good option after surgery or radiation because penile deterioration occurs by waiting and men should start a treatment 3 months after prostate cancer therapy.

Impotence, or erectile dysfunction, is the inability to achieve or maintain an erection of sufficient girth and rigidity long enough for penetration and intercourse. It is not the same as loss of libido or sex drive, which may be caused by hormonal therapy, although loss of libido may be a natural occurrence if a man knows he is unable to get an erection. Although we commonly believe that first a man gets aroused and then he gets an erection, it very often works the other way. An erect penis will stimulate and improve libido. It is not uncommon for men to complain that they have lost their libido or desire for sex when they are no longer having erections.

Prostate cancer is not the only cause of impotence. About one in 10 men becomes impotent as a result of health problems such as diabetes, high blood pressure, spinal cord injuries, and even certain medications. The National Institutes of Health estimate that from 10 to 20 million men in the United States between the ages of 40 and 70 suffer erectile dysfunction, but less than 10 percent do anything about it. Indeed, many men simply assume it is a condition of aging and do not realize it is a medical condition that can be treated.

Your wife or intimate partner needs to be fully involved in learning about and helping you decide on treatment, and both of you should talk with your physician about your options. Affection and intimacy are important during recovery, and while you and your partner are adapting, it may take some trial and error to see whether Muse (see page 172), or penile injections, or a vacuum device suits you and to evaluate the effect they have on your ability to make love. Some men say the vacuum device makes their penis feel cold; others say the injection makes it feel artificial. There are also many false assumptions about penile prostheses, including a belief that it requires a pump that is located outside the scrotum. Sometimes in an effort to be supportive women discourage their partner from considering a prosthesis because they believe it is dangerous and that there are other ways to make love. However, they may not understand the deeper psychological reasons a man needs to maintain his self-image as a man. Each man and his partner are individuals and they need to find what is best for them.

The Mechanics of an Erection

Explanations of how a penis becomes erect have been revised over time, but it is generally believed that the blood circulation changes when a man is aroused by physical or psychological means. The increased blood flow causes spaces in the penis filled with spongy tissue to expand. These spongy areas run along the length of the penis on the right and left sides. When the brain lets the penis know about sexual arousal, the erection begins. Nerves relax the blood vessels in the spongy tissue so that more blood can get in. As these spongy tissues fill with blood and become engorged, they press against veins that normally take blood out of the penis. The blood becomes trapped in the penis and an erection results.

The veins, arteries, and nerves must be intact and healthy to achieve and maintain an erection. After radical surgery or radiation therapy, most of these nerves and blood vessels may become injured and may not function properly, resulting in erectile dysfunction.

Treatment Options

There are many new and improved therapies available to correct erectile dysfunction. It is possible to continue having sexual intercourse with the help of medications injected into the penis or inserted into the urethra, implanted penile prostheses, or a vacuum erection device. As this book is written, new drugs are being studied and it may soon be possible to take a pill to have an erection.

Urologists specializing in sexual dysfunction are available in most major medical centers. There are more than 40 such centers around the United States that specialize in correcting erectile dysfunction with the penile injection system.

There are sex therapists who can counsel about the emotional aspects of sexual dysfunction, but it is important to check their credentials first and to question how they have helped other men and how many men have continued to enjoy their sex lives using such treatment plans.

Books and videos are available through doctors, drug companies, and the penile device manufacturers. These materials can help you and your partner learn how to practice new methods for restoring sex to your lives.

Appendix 1 has a list of organizations that can help you start your search for information. The American Cancer Society has an excellent free booklet about sexuality after cancer treatment. Call your local branch to get a copy of *Sexuality and Cancer: For the Man Who Has Cancer and His Partner.*

Vacuum Erection Device (VED)

This simple mechanical device has a cylinder, pump, and rubber band. The cylinder fits over the penis, and when air is pumped out, a partial vacuum is created. The vacuum draws blood into the penis so that an erection can be achieved. The blood is trapped in the penis by slipping an elastic band over the base.

The results differ somewhat from a normal erection. For example, the penis may feel slightly cold. It may be larger in circumference and it will pivot at the base. The penis will not be as stiff at the base but may be very hard at the end. Veins may be distended and it may look blue. Sometimes men notice a numbness while the constriction is in place, but this does not usually decrease pleasure. Some men find it easier to reach orgasm when they use the device, but a few find it more difficult.

An advantage of the vacuum device is that it mimics the natural process and allows complete control of when you want the erection to begin and end. Some men and their partners believe it is better than nothing, whereas others say it seems mechanical and artificial. The major disadvantage, however, is that time is taken away from foreplay to use the pump, and some men and their partners feel that this can be disruptive. It may also worsen incontinence.

The vacuum device is not considered the best treatment option, especially for younger men who have had surgery. The following options may have more to offer.

Transurethral Therapy

In 1996, the FDA approved a new drug called Muse, a medicated pellet that can be inserted directly into the urethra through the penis. The medication diffuses into the erectile bodies of the penis to cause dilation of the blood vessels and thus an erection. Erection occurs about 5 to 10 minutes after application.

This drug is similar to that used for penile injections, but the dosage is greater and thus the side effects may be more pronounced. The introduction of Muse is the first time that alprostadil, a synthetic prostaglandin, can be used in the treatment of erectile dysfunction without having to inject it. It comes in a prefilled plastic applicator with a suppository of the drug to be dropped into the urethra. It is available in four dosages from 125 to 1,000 micrograms. Lower doses are usually prescribed in the beginning. It is not a good idea to use this system more than twice in a 24-hour period.

From what has been observed in a short amount of time, Muse seems to work in only a small percentage of men after a radical prostatectomy. About 25 percent will obtain partial erections adequate for intercourse, but the majority do not respond. Over half of men who use Muse complain of a mild to modest penile pain. Some men will adapt to the pain, but many cannot tolerate it. It seems to work better for men who can almost get an erection but who need a boost to augment the limited erection they can achieve on their own.

The medicated pellet comes with an applicator to help push the pellet about an inch or two into the urethra. This can be done sitting or standing and stretching the penis slowly upward to its full length and gently squeezing on the glans (the head of the penis) to open the urethra. While the penis is stretched, the applicator stem can be inserted into the urethra. When a button on the applicator is pushed, the medication will drop into the urethra. Rocking the applicator from side to side assures that the pellet gets into the urethra.

Then, keeping the penis extended to its full length, it should be rolled between the hands for a few seconds to ensure that the medication is properly absorbed along the walls of the urethra so that it can get to the blood vessels. For a man with a curved or unnaturally shaped penis, this drug may not be safe. Its effectiveness is based on a straight penis and urethra so that the drug can pass all the way through the length of the penis.

After the drug has been administered, it is important not to sit or lie down for at least 10 minutes. Walking around increases the blood flow to the penis and provides a better erection. An erection should last from 30 minutes to an hour.

Many patients need to experiment with different dosages before satisfaction is achieved. Men with hypertension, sickle cell disease, abnormal penile anatomy, or with other conditions that predispose to priapism, and in whom sexual activity is not advised, should not use Muse. It should not be used if your partner is pregnant unless you use a condom.

Side Effects of Transurethral Therapy

All vasodilators can cause side effects in some men. Some of these drugs can produce a painful, prolonged erection known as priapism that requires immediate medical attention if it lasts more than 4 hours. Priapism is usually caused by too large a dose of the medication. With proper education and testing in the doctor's office, the correct amount of drug will be prescribed and priapism can be avoided.

Because the Muse uses a much larger dose of alprostadil than the penile injection therapy, it also has more side effects in the surrounding and distal tissues of the penis. For instance, patients who have varicose veins will experience dilation of their varicose veins even though the veins are far away from the penis. This does not happen with penile injections.

Muse is a new therapy and there are no long-term studies of its effectiveness and the side effects. However, the most common side effects, other than priapism, observed in clinical trials of the medicated pellet are:

- Mild to moderate penile pain (the most frequently reported side effect)
- Burning or warmth in the urethra
- Redness of the penis from the increased blood flow
- Some urethral bleeding or spotting if the drug is not administered properly
- Some vaginal itching or burning reported by female partners

Other very rare side effects include dizziness or headache, rapid pulse, and an increase in liver enzymes. Injecting medication can be painful.

Pharmacologic Erection Program (PEP)

The same type of medication used for the transurethral therapy is used by injection directly into the penis. The penile injection system initially requires training and monitoring by a physician. Two office visits designed to teach you how to give yourself the injections and test your response to the drug are generally needed. Finding the correct dosage is vitally important. Too little will not be effective and too much could cause an erection to last too long and become painful. During initial testing, the urologist may use the Doppler ultrasound test to scan your penis in its flaccid state and then again after an injection, to measure the arterial blood flow and note the difference in diameter of the dilated penile artery. Then you will get a prescription for kits with disposable sterile syringes and needles.

The largest study of penile injections was done by the Department of Urology at New York Hospital–Cornell Medical Center from 1988 to 1996. More than 1,000 patients were enrolled in the pharmacological erection program and investigators studied the predictors of success and risk factors for attrition. Men who discontinued the therapy dropped out within the first 2 months, and the attrition rate for the next 2 years was less than 10 percent. Among those who stopped the therapy, more than half received penile prostheses. The study suggests that doctors carefully counsel their patients, especially during the early months of therapy, to help them use it successfully or find a better therapy such as penile prosthesis.

Before you consider using the penile injection system, consider your own manual dexterity, your past medical history, and genital anatomy. Some men say it is unnatural and they or their partners are afraid to touch their penis. Others claim they felt they were not in control. This system will not be appropriate for you if you have poor vision or poor manual dexterity and if you are unwilling to follow instructions.

Injecting Yourself

The kit comes with everything you need for a treatment: a vial of medication called Caverject, a syringe, a needle, and alcohol swabs. The vials come in strengths of 10 or 20 micrograms and are for one-time use only.

Wash your hands and set out the items from the package on a clean surface. Assemble the syringe, remove the cap, and swab the stopper with alcohol. Remove the needle guard, and holding the needle pointed toward the ceiling, push the plunger into the syringe to force the air out. Then push the needle into the vial of medication and swirl the medication around. Pull the plunger back and the medication will fill the syringe. If you see air bubbles inside the syringe, just tap it gently and the bubbles will burst as air leaves the syringe.

Always alternate injections on the left and right side of your penis so that you don't irritate one side and to minimize scarring. Retract the foreskin, and avoiding veins, hold the needle at a 90-degree angle with the shaft of your penis. The needle is short and you may feel a pinch, but there is little pain. You should have an erection in 5 to 20 minutes after injection. It should last for 45 minutes to an hour. If it lasts too long, your physician will lower the medication dosage.

It is important to visit your physician every 3 months to review your technique and to have your penis examined to be sure there are no obvious side effects. Injections should not exceed 12 a month and it is best if they are evenly spaced.

Side Effects of Penile Injections

In addition to side effects of the medication itself described in the information about Muse, there are two types of potential side effects of the penile injection program. One is simply that whenever a needle is stuck in the body a bruise can develop. Over time a small nodule or lump may occur due to injecting again and again in the same site. Also extremely rare is a slight dull ache in the penis, but this usually subsides after about 15 minutes.

Penile Prostheses

For some men, a penile prosthesis can be the most satisfactory way to restore potency, and some men have said they like it so well that they never want their old penis back. The main advantage is that an erection can be maintained for as long as you need it. Many men also continue to have a spontaneous partial erection with the penile prosthesis.

There are several types of prostheses. Some are made of silicone and some of a synthetic rubberlike material called elastomer. Some are made of both. The fluid used is generally saline—a saltwater solution that cannot harm the body if it should leak out of the prosthesis. Penile prostheses adapt well to the body and have a very low risk of infection. Mechanical failure is the most significant problem, and some prostheses need to be replaced when they wear out.

• The malleable-type prosthesis is the easiest to implant. Two semirigid rods are implanted into the penis, which will then always be erect. It is simply bent down to conceal it and raised when needed.

• The two-cylinder prosthesis can leave the penis erect or flaccid. A hardening agent is transferred from one cylinder in the penis to the other when the prosthesis is activated. This is done by squeezing the head of the penis where the pump is located. Fluid is then released into the other cylinder to make the penis erect. To turn off the erection, the penis can simply be bent downward and the fluid will leave the penile cylinder and return to the storage cylinder.

• The fully inflatable device is the most expensive and complex, but also the most natural. Inflatable cylinders are implanted into the penis, and the reservoir of fluid is implanted in the lower abdomen. This reservoir can be implanted at the same time as a prostatectomy is performed.

Surgical Implantation

All prostheses can be surgically implanted using local or regional anesthesia, and most patients go home by the next day. Some pain or discomfort may be apparent for several days until the surgery heals. The first erection can be painful, but this discomfort is temporary.

Men often have the reservoir implanted at the time of their prostatectomy so that they will not need additional surgery later. If they eventually find that they do not need the prosthesis, then the reservoir can simply remain in place without causing any harm.

This procedure must be performed by someone who does a large volume of such implants. It takes a long time to learn this surgery and remain proficient. A surgeon should do at least 30 to 40 penile prostheses a year to maintain the necessary level of skill. If the surgeon does less than 10 a year, it is very unlikely the results will be good.

The Cost of Treatment

Treatment for erectile dysfunction can be expensive but is generally covered by medical insurance. A vacuum device costs from $400 to $500 depending on whether you get the battery-assisted model or manual unit. It is covered by Medicare and most other insurance plans. Penile injections cost anywhere from $10 to $25 per injection depending on the medication used. It may cost about $200 for a 2-month supply of drugs and syringes plus doctor visits. Penile implants, requiring surgery, are naturally more costly.

19

Monitoring Your Health

In the 2 years following surgery or radiation treatment for prostate cancer you will need to visit your urologist and possibly your radiation therapist every 3 months for a checkup. After that, 6-month checkups will be required. Regularly scheduled checkups are mandatory! Once you have had cancer, you are at increased risk for disease recurrence or progression, so surveillance becomes a way of life. The urologist will monitor your prostate cancer for the rest of your life and it is important to keep your regularly scheduled visits so that any checkups or tests are done at appropriate intervals.

If you have had radiation therapy, your radiation oncologist may want to examine you periodically following treatment to monitor for any side effects or recurrence. Your primary follow-up care will generally be with your urologist.

While your urologist is keeping tabs on your prostate cancer, your overall health needs the attention of your primary care physician. An annual physical checkup should be part of your routine and should include a DRE with fecal occult blood test and chest X-ray. Other tests and lab work depend on your age and condition. Keep your family doctor well informed about your follow-up care with the prostate cancer treatment team, such as blood test results from your urologist. If you don't have a family doctor or primary care physician, this may be a good time to find one.

PSA Surveillance

PSA is the primary surveillance tool to watch for the recurrence of prostate cancer. After treatment the PSA should drop to low levels and stay there, but once again, age, race, and the treatment you had will have an effect. The PSA level can become a source of anxiety for men because they naturally don't want to see it rise. Some more obsessive men will plot their PSA results over time and will surf the Internet looking for meaning to their numbers and curves. But the PSA, like the stock market, is not an absolute. The PSA values may suggest trends but cannot be used with certainty to predict the future.

Without a Prostate, How Can There Be PSA?

Theoretically, once the prostate—and the cancer—is removed, your PSA should drop down to the lowest possible level for your age and race. It normally takes a few weeks for the remaining PSA to leave your system. This does not always happen. Microscopic prostate epithelial cells can remain in the prostate bed and continue to produce PSA. It could take 5 or more years for microscopic tumor cells lurking in the prostate bed to grow enough to produce PSA that will be detectable.

If metastasis was unrecognized prior to treatment for cancer presumed to be localized, the PSA will rise fairly quickly. But if the cancer recurs locally after treatment, the rise in PSA may take longer—as much as 5 or 10 years. You cannot be lulled into a false sense of security. You need to monitor the PSA for the rest of your life.

By now you probably know a great deal more about PSA than before your treatment, but because this is such an important indicator, it needs to be reviewed and put into perspective. What should you expect after surgery? After radiation? While you are being treated with hormones?

After treatment, try to be cautiously optimistic. If the PSA level rises, you need to find out why. Was it because not all the cancer was killed by the radiation? Was there undetected cancer before surgery located outside the prostate, perhaps in the bones or lymph nodes?

As stated throughout this book, there is no absolute. Your PSA must be measured in context with your age, race, and medical condition. If your PSA was high before you discovered prostate cancer, it does not automatically mean the cause was cancer. You may have had benign prostatic hyperplasia (BPH) or prostatitis. But once you are known to have prostate cancer, the increases in the PSA level are more likely to be cause for concern. If your prostate was surgically removed, then you cannot have BPH or prostatitis.

If your PSA is suddenly higher, have the test repeated. There is always a chance for laboratory error. There are other reasons it could rise. For example, if you have your blood tested within 24 hours of ejaculation, your PSA will be up. If you ride a bike for any length of time, that could also cause the level to rise.

The PSA level varies during and after certain types of treatment. For example, after being treated with finasteride (Proscar), for symptomatic BPH, the PSA level drops, but it is an artificial response to the drug. Anyone taking this drug is advised by his physician to double the PSA to estimate the true value.

Your PSA can be considered something of a magic marker. It will let you know if your cancer has been effectively treated or whether there may be a sign of metastasis or local recurrence. Although the PSA test is not 100 percent effective by itself as a screening tool to find prostate cancer, it is a remarkable tool for monitoring the presence or absence of prostate cancer once you have had treatment for the disease. You will probably need to check your PSA every 3 months for the first year. If your cancer was detected early and you had curative treatment with surgery or radiation, your PSA may remain in the undetectable range forever.

Pay attention to signals from your body such as persistent pain in your lower back, which might indicate bone metastasis. Increased urinary symptoms or blood in the urine could indicate recurrence. Never hesitate to bring anything to your doctor's attention. If it turns out not to be important, then you will feel better and your doctor will know that you are paying attention to your health.

We have no long-term studies with meaningful data on prostate cancer recurrence rates after surgery or radiation treatment. Because prostate cancer grows slowly, researchers need at least 15 years to determine if a treatment is effective. A 1992 study found that when cancer did not escape the confines of the prostate, only 2 percent of men had local recurrences within 5 years after radical prostatectomy and 1 percent had distant metastases. A Medicare survey of older men showed 28 percent to have recurrence after radical prostatectomy. Overall, the recurrence rate is 12 percent.

Although no long-term studies are completed about survival rates for internal or external radiation treatment, the early reports look encouraging. Five-year follow-up studies indicate that radiation therapy is as effective as radical prostatectomy in curing localized prostate cancer.

What to Expect

If you had a prostatectomy, the first PSA test will probably be done a month after surgery, generally 2 weeks after the catheter is removed. This protocol is determined by what we know about the half-life of the PSA. Half-life is the time taken for the PSA level to drop by half, say from 6 to 3. PSA has a half-life of 2 to 3 days, and it generally takes 5 half-lives for PSA to leave your system after surgery. Therefore, a month after surgery is when a new PSA reading would tell us something meaningful.

If PSA remains high or rises soon after surgery, it could mean the disease has already metastasized and this was not recognized prior to surgery. If it rises later, after a period of months to years, it may suggest a local recurrence of the cancer in the bed where the prostate used to be.

Following radiation therapy, PSA should gradually fall to low levels within a year. If it drops to less than 1.0, the cancer has probably been effectively treated. If it stays above 2.0 after a year, there may still be some cancer present.

Most recent radical prostatectomy and radiation studies suggest that testing PSA levels after treatment is the most sensitive way to know if treatment has achieved effective local control or not. Following surgery, for example, an absolute PSA value should approach 0.1 or less. However, most surgical studies use cutoff points from 0.3 to 0.6. Most studies reporting results of external beam radiation and brachytherapy have been arbitrarily set to a PSA of less than 4.0. Several reports suggest that achievement of PSA nadir less than 1.0 is an important predictor of treatment success. But there is no absolute consensus.

Once you have been diagnosed with prostate cancer, the PSA becomes a very important yardstick for monitoring the effects of treatment on the progress of the disease. You need to keep tabs on your PSA and know what it is doing for the rest of your life.

Maintaining Vigilance

If your PSA rises and your doctor suspects it is due to a recurrence of your cancer, then other diagnostic tests can confirm this suspicion or rule it out. A transrectal sonogram or CAT scan will examine the immediate area of the prostate or the prostate bed. A bone scan will look for bone metastasis. (Refer to Chapter 5 for more information about diagnostic testing.)

Nobody knows if a cancer will recur. We can only calculate the odds based on everything we learn through diagnosis and treatment. By understanding tumor volume, cell activity, lymph node status, and staging, we can estimate that someone has a 10 percent chance of recurrence or a 65 percent chance, but this does not mean that the cancer will recur. Nor is there any guarantee that someone won't have a recurrence even with only a 5 percent chance.

Recurrence can be:

- Local—reappearance at the same site (prostate bed, seminal vesicles)
- Regional—reappearance near the original site (lymph nodes)
- Metastatic—reappearance elsewhere in the body (bone)

Despite the lack of definitive long-term studies of 15 years or more, a study at Stanford University of 1,400 men with T1 or T2 disease who had radical prostatectomy has given us some idea about what to expect. If the cancer was in the prostate transition zone (the area surrounding the hole of the doughnut), there is an 80 percent cure rate with radical prostatectomy. If the cancer was in the peripheral zone, the cure rate drops to 53 percent. In 38 percent of all men studied, the PSA rate never dropped after surgery, so the cancer had already metastasized but was not recognized before surgery. There was a 19 percent failure rate after 1 year, 26 percent after 2 years, and 2 percent after 5 years.

Staying Healthy

After treatment for prostate cancer or any problems with their prostate, Chinese patients often ask, "How can I change my diet so that I will stay healthy?" This question, an intriguing one, is less often asked by American men. Eating well and getting regular exercise, as well as getting rid of some of the stress in your life, can do a lot to prolong your life. Although it is not possible to point to one food or type of exercise and say it will prevent cancer, many studies suggest that nutrition and exercise can contribute to keeping your body (and mind) fit, and a fit body does not succumb to illness as easily as one that is out of shape.

Whether you expect to live for many years or your life expectancy has been shortened by disease, you can live the best you can. If you eat well, exercise, and take care of your health, you may feel even better than you did before.

Reducing Your Fat Consumption

Cutting out the fat is not easy. Fat, like salt and sugar, is addictive, and it may take a while to withdraw. You may not be able to go cold turkey. When you try to curb your hunger with a carrot rather than a bowl of ice cream, your fat cells will be screaming for satisfaction.

Start by cutting back on the obvious—red meat, fried foods, excess butter and eggs, whole milk, ice cream. Make it a practice to read labels on packaged foods and avoid those with a high percentage of fat. Look for an inexpensive pocket guide to calories and fat grams available in most bookstores. Many are available free from health agencies such as the American Cancer Society and the American Heart Association.

A 1996 Harris poll concluded that 74 percent of Americans are overweight. About a third of adult Americans are so overweight that they are obese according to the U.S. Census Bureau. Approximately 58 million adults in the United States are overweight and the number is growing. Being overweight means being more than 20 percent over your ideal weight, and obesity is defined as being 40 percent over your ideal weight. The rate of obesity has risen from 25 percent of the population in 1980 to 33.4 percent in 1991.

Few of us need more than 2,000 calories a day, yet 3,700 is closer to the daily average American diet. According to the American Cancer Society, the risk of getting cancer increases 2.3 percent for each 100 calories per day over the recommended amount.

Exercising

It will take a while after surgery to feel like walking to the corner, never mind run a marathon, but do get moving as soon as you feel up to it. Exercise strengthens your heart and lungs and lifts your spirits.

Try to make exercise directed toward muscle strengthening and cardiovascular fitness part of your daily routine. Walking is one of the best cardiovascular exercises. Walking every day for half an hour will help you stay fit. Walk as quickly as you can with your arms swinging. Start slowly but let it become part of your life. Once your body gets used to exercising, it will crave it and a good habit will develop. You need at least 20 minutes of vigorous exercise three times a week. If you exercise longer than 20 minutes at a time, you'll start to burn off calories.

If you have access to a health club or YMCA, that's a good beginning. People of all ages and conditions participate in fitness programs these days. Treadmills, bicycles, stair machines, and rowing machines are all metered to tell you how much work you are doing. The best machines for cardiovascular fitness put your large muscles in motion.

The Future for You and Your Family

It is important to talk with your male relatives and encourage them to get regular screening tests for prostate cancer. If you have a son, he should begin early screening at age 40 because his risk could be higher since his father had cancer. Share your prostate cancer history and encourage relatives to share it with their own doctors so that they will be diligent about getting regular DREs and PSAs. Urge your friends to be aware of how to prevent a disease that does not have to take so many lives.

Lahey Hitchcock Clinic in Burlington, Massachusetts, is conducting a 5-year study to identify the hereditary link in families with multiple cases of prostate cancer. If you have at least one other blood relative with prostate cancer and at least one of you is living with or has survived the cancer, you are eligible to participate in this study. There is no need to travel anywhere or take any tests other than a blood test. For information, call the Hereditary Prostate Cancer Project at 1-800-348-8855 between 8 A.M. and 5 P.M. eastern standard time.

Hopefully, as treatment improves, as doctors learn how to educate their patients as well as care for them, as patients take more responsibility for their care, as preventive health care becomes more widespread, and as health insurance becomes more accessible and affordable, we can wipe out prostate cancer. In the meantime, carry the message with you. Early detection is the cure.

Every day medical science learns more about treating cancer, but we hope that in our lifetime we will no longer have to treat it—we will be able to prevent it. Some truly exciting and hopeful research studies are in progress as we end this book.

Immunotherapy looks like the most hopeful way to finally cure cancer and we may be only a few years away. We will be able to make the immune system recognize cancer as an agent that it must destroy the same way it destroys bacteria and germs and other foreign bodies that enter the system.

In this age of dramatic advancement in biomolecular knowledge, our chances of finding a cure have increased enormously.

We hope you find this book helpful and we hope you take our advice: Get the best treatment you can and take good care of yourself.

Appendix 1

Information Resources

A wide network of information resources about prostate cancer is available. People who answer telephone hotlines are specially trained to provide up-to-date information and most of these agencies can provide the information in Spanish as well as English (occasionally in other languages). If you call with a question or need a referral, they can help you. If they can't help, they will know who can.

NCI Cancer Information Service Hotline
1-800-4-CANCER (1-800-422-6237)

The National Cancer Institute (NCI) is the primary federal agency for cancer research and information on everything from clinical trials to new drugs. The hotline is operated by a network of authorized comprehensive cancer centers, and you'll be connected with the one nearest you. NCI keeps an up-to-date file of available resources and physicians. The hotline operates weekdays from 9 A.M. to 4:30 P.M. eastern standard time.

Material is from PDQ, a computer service that gives up-to-date information on cancer treatment. It is a service for people with cancer and their families, and for doctors, nurses, and other health care professionals. PDQ information is reviewed each month by cancer experts and is updated when the information changes. PDQ also lists information about research on new treatments, clinical trials, doctors who treat cancer, and hospitals with cancer programs.

You can also obtain information from NCI by fax or through the Internet.

• **CancerFax (301-402-5874)** is a way to obtain PDQ information statements in English or Spanish using a fax machine. It contains fact sheets on various cancer topics from NCI's office of cancer communications. CancerFax operates 24 hours a day, 7 days a week, with no other charge than the telephone call. For a fact sheet explaining how to use CancerFax, call 1-800-4-CANCER.

• **CancerNet** at **cancernet@icicc.nci.nih.gov** and enter the word HELP in the BODY of the mail message. (The information is also available in Spanish.) CancerNet will send you a return mail message containing the contents list of materials available through CancerNet. There is no charge.

American Cancer Society
1-800-ACS-2345 (1-800-227-2345) for your local chapter
(http://www.cancer.org/proearly.html)

With 3,400 chapters in the United States, ACS is the largest voluntary health agency in the world. ACS sponsors research, education, and patient service programs, including transportation to and from treatment, support groups, and equipment loans. It is usually a good way to find out what resources are available in your community. ACS has affiliated programs:

• **Man to Man.** Prostate cancer support groups as well as a one-on-one visitation program for men who do not feel comfortable discussing their concerns in a group setting are available. Specially trained volunteers who are prostate cancer survivors themselves talk with you in your home, at the hospital, or over the phone. This program does not give medical advice but rather support for men going through treatments for prostate cancer.

There is also a Man to Man network on the Internet, designed primarily to provide education about prostate cancer and let men know that they can get help by seeking out support systems and other survivors.

• **Man to Man Prostate Cancer Education and Support subsite on the World Wide Web home page (http://www.cancer.org).** Here you can find background information about the Man to Man program, general information about the PSA blood tests, incontinence, and an interview with author Michael Korda, who wrote a book about his experience with prostate cancer.

Us Too! International, Inc. Toll-free hotline:
1-800-80-USTOO (1-800-808-7866)
930 North York Road, Suite 50
Hinsdale, IL 60521-2993
708-323-1002
708-323-1003 (fax)

Organized in 1990 by men with prostate cancer who wanted help in deciding on treatment options, this very strong advocacy and support network has chapters in all parts of the world. There are more than 500 chapters in Europe, Africa, Japan, South America, the Middle East, and Asia. Most are managed by volunteer regional directors. The group publishes a newsletter.

Internet addresses: www.ustoo.com.

For general information about prostate cancer and support group information.

Home page of Mediconsult.com. Access at
http://www.prostate.com.

For the Us Too newsletter, *Prostate Cancer Communicator.*

Cancer Care
National toll-free counseling line
1-800-813-HOPE   (1-800-813-4673)
1180 Avenue of the Americas
New York, NY 10036
212-221-3300

Cancer Care is a voluntary agency, founded in 1944, dedicated to providing support for cancer patients and their families and friends, as well as education for the general public. It offers professional social work counseling and guidance free of charge and serves about 50,000 people a year. Cancer Care focuses on helping cancer patients at any stage of illness to cope with the emotional, social, and financial burdens of cancer.

Financial assistance of nearly $1.4 million is provided annually to eligible families to help with home care, transportation, pain medication, and medical treatment costs.

A nationwide counseling line—offered in English, Spanish, and Yiddish—provides emotional support, problem solving, and guidance with doctors—patient communication, second opinions, finding your way through the health care system, information and referral to local community resources, and a computerized resource directory. Practical guidelines for obtaining home care, transportation to treatment, and access to entitlements are also provided.

Programs of professional consultation and education, community education and awareness, social research, and public policy are conducted on a local and national level. Cancer Care provides free education materials on a range of cancer diagnoses and treatment options. Telephone support groups and educational seminars are available for patients, family members, and caregivers.

National Coalition for Cancer Survivorship (NCCS)
1010 Wayne Avenue, Suite 300
Silver Spring, MD 20910
301-585-2616
http://www.access.digex.net

This network of independent groups and individuals is concerned with survivorship and support of cancer survivors and their loved ones. NCCS's primary goal is to promote a national awareness of issues affecting cancer survivors. Its objectives are to serve as a clearinghouse for information on services and materials for survivors, advocate the rights and interests of cancer survivors, encourage the study of survivorship, and promote the development of cancer support activities.

American College of Surgeons Committee on Cancer
55 East Erie St.
Chicago, IL 60611
http://www.facs.org/public.info/ppserv.html

Write for a booklet listing approved cancer programs. Revised quarterly.

The Prostate Health Council
American Federation for Urologic Disease (AFUD)
300 West Pratt Street, Suite 401
Baltimore, MD 21201
1-800-242-2383 for information
1-800-7866 for support group network

A great resource for patients with urological conditions including benign prostatic hyperplasia (BPH), prostate cancer, impotence, and infertility.

National Kidney and Urologic Diseases Information Clearinghouse
P.O. Box NKUDIC
9000 Rockville Pike
Bethesda, MD 20892
http://www.aerie.com/nihdb/nkudic/kudbase.html

Ask for information on impotence and incontinence.

American Urological Association
1120 North Charles Street
Baltimore, MD 21201
410-727-1100
http://www.ananet.org/

CaP Cure
1250 Fourth Street, Suite 360
Santa Monica, CA 90401
310-458-2873
http://www.capcure.org/

For Help with Incontinence

The following organizations can give you information about groups in your area where you can get more information, help from support groups, educational and emotional support.

Home Delivery Incontinent
1-800-538-1036

National Association for Continence (NAFC)
P.O. Box 544
Union, SC 29379
803-579-7900
http://www.nafc.org/

For Help with Impotence

American Association of Sex Educators, Counselors and Therapists (AASECT)
11 Dupont Circle, NW, Suite 220
Washington, DC 20036
202-462-1171

Offers assistance in finding a sex therapist.

Sex Information and Education Council of the U.S. (SIECUS)
130 West 42nd Street, Suite 350
New York, NY 10036
212-819-9770
http://www.siecus.org/

Impotence Information Center
P.O. Box 9, Dept. USA
Minneapolis, MN 55440
1-800-843-4615

Offers help finding a support group in your area.

Impotence Anonymous
119 S. Ruth St., Box 1257
Maryville, TN 37801-5743
615-983-6064

This group has chapters throughout the United States. Send a stamped self-addressed envelope for list of chapters.

Potency Restored
c/o Giulio Scarzella, MD
8630 Fenton Street, Suite 218
Silver Spring, MD 10910

Write for information about chapters in many states.

Recovery of Male Potency (ROMP)
c/o Grace Hospital
18700 Meyers Road
Detroit, MI 48235
1-800-TEL-ROMP outside Michigan
313-927-3219 for Michigan residents

ROMP has chapters in many states.

Not for Men Only
c/o Mercy Hospital and Medical Center
Stevenson Expressway at King Drive
Chicago, IL 60616
1-800-448-8664 outside Chicago
312-567-5567 in Illinois

Groups for couples as well as groups for men or women.

Impotence Institute of America
10400 Little Patuxent Parkway, Suite 485
Columbia, MD 21044-3502
1-800-669-1603

Erectile Dysfunction Unit
New York Hospital–Cornell Medical Center
428 East 72nd Street
New York, NY 10021
212-746-5473

Appendix 2

Selected Studies

Epidemiologic Characteristics of Prostate Cancer
Edward Giovannucci, MD, ScD, Department of Medicine, Harvard
    Medical School and Brigham and Women's Hospital, Boston, Mas-
    sachusetts
Cancer Supplement, Volume 75, No. 7, April 1, 1995
Presented at the National Conference on Prostate Cancer, Philadelphia,
PA, September 29 to October 1, 1994

Studies on soy and tomatoes reported by Giovannucci, a researcher at
the Harvard School of Public Health, in the *Journal of the National Cancer
Institute,* December 7, 1995, 9-year study of eating habits of 47,000 men

**Decreased Growth of Established Human Prostate LNCaP
Tumors in Nude Mice Fed a Low-Fat Diet**
Yu Wang, John G. Corr, Howard T. Thaler, Ue Tao, William R. Fair,
    Warren D. W. Heston, all of Memorial Sloan-Kettering Cancer Cen-
    ter
Journal of the National Cancer Institute, Vol. 87, No. 19, October 4, 1995

Dietary Fat, Fatty Acids and Prostate Cancer
David P. Rose and Jeanne M. Connolly
Division of Nutrition and Endocrinology, American Health Foundation
Lipids, Vol. 27, No. 10, 1992

**Family History and Prostate Cancer Risk in Black, White,
and Asian Men in the United States and Canada**
Whittlemore, Wu, Kolonal, John, Gallagher, Howe, West, Ten, Stamey,
    The Johns Hopkins University School of Hygiene and Public Health
American Journal of Epidemiology, Vol. 141, No. 8, 1995

**Comparative Epidemiology of Cancers of the Colon,
Rectum, Prostate and Breast in Shanghai China versus the
United States**

Yu, Harris, Gao, Gao, Wyndner, The American Health Foundation, Shanghai Cancer Institute, Ohio State University Department of Preventive Medicine
International Journal of Epidemiology, Vol. 20, No. 1, 1991

Does the Racial-Ethnic Variation in Prostate Cancer Risk Have a Hormonal Basis?
Ronald K. Ross, MD, Gerhard Coetzee, Ph.D., Juergen Reichardt, Ph.D., Eila Skinner, MD, Brian Henderson, MD, University of Southern California, and the Salk Institute
Cancer Supplement, Vol. 75, No. 7, April 1, 1995
Presented September 29 to October 1, 1994, National Conference on Prostate Cancer, Philadelphia, PA

A Double-Blind Clinical Trial of the Effects of Soy Protein on Risk Parameters for Prostate Cancer
Barnes, Urban, Grizzle, Coward, Kirk, Weiss, Irwin, Comprehensive Cancer Center, University of Alabama at Birmingham, 1996–1997

Statistical Comparison of Progression-free Likelihood
Walsh and Partin, 1994, The Johns Hopkins University School of Medicine
Comparison of 561 men at Johns Hopkins University Hospital who were subjected to staging pelvic lymphadenectomy with or without radical prostatectomy from 1975 to 1987, and the series of Johansson et al. and Fuks et al. from *Campbell's Urology*, 6th edition.

Results of Radical Prostatectomy in Men with Clinically Localized Prostate Cancer
Gerber et al., a multi-institutional pooled analysis, University of Chicago, Baylor College of Medicine, University of Wurzburg (Germany), Erasmus University (Netherlands), Duke University School of Medicine, University of Utah School of Medicine, Vanderbilt University School of Medicine, Eastern Virginia Medical School
Journal of the American Medical Association, Vol. 276, No. 8, August 28, 1996

Study of Medicare Patients from 1984 to 1990
Grace L. Lu-Yao, Dartmouth Medical School

Ongoing Study to Determine the Long-term Effectiveness of Thwarting Prostate Cancer with Seed Therapy

Dr. Kent Wallner and colleagues, Department of Radiation–Oncology, Memorial Sloan-Kettering Cancer Center

Defining the Role of Antiandrogens in the Treatment of Prostate Cancer

David G. McLeod, MD, JD, and Geert J. C. M. Kolvenbag, MD, Walter Reed Army Medical Center, Uniformed Services University of the Health Sciences, and Zeneca Pharmaceuticals

Urology, January 1996

Hormone Therapy for Prostate Cancer: A Topical Perspective

Eric A. Klein, MD, The Cleveland Clinic Foundation, and Zeneca Pharmaceuticals

Urology, January 1996

Predictors of Success and Risk Factors for Attrition in the Use of Intracavernous Injection

Ruchira Gupta, Jill Kirschen, Robert C. Barrow, II, and Jean François Eid, Department of Urology, New York Hospital–Cornell Medical Center

Journal of Urology, Vol. 157, pp. 1681–1686, May 1997

Appendix 3

Bibliography

You can find many books in your library or bookstore about prostate cancer and there are also videos on the subject that can be borrowed or rented from libraries or from your physician or the hospital patient education department. Because protocols for treating prostate cancer are changing, no book published before 1995 is listed. Here are two suggested books to review.

Korda, Michael. *Man to Man: Surviving Prostate Cancer.* Random House, New York, 1996.

Walsh, Patrick, M.D., and Janet Farrar Worthington. *The Prostate: A Guide for Men and the Women Who Love Them.* Johns Hopkins University Press, Baltimore, 1995.

Free Publications

Facing Forward: A Guide for Cancer Survivors. NIH Publication No. 93-2424. Free 43-page booklet from the National Institutes of Health, National Cancer Institute. Revised October 1992. Good solid information on continuing your health care after cancer, managing insurance issues, confronting your feelings, earning a living, and moving ahead.

National Cancer Institute (NCI)
9000 Rockville Pike
Bethesda, MD 20892

Other publications from NCI:
What You Need to Know About Prostate Cancer
Radiation Therapy and You
What Are Clinical Trials All About?

Patient to Patient: Cancer Clinical Trials and You
Taking Time: Support for People with Cancer and the People Who Care About Them
When Cancer Recurs: Meeting the Challenge Again
Advanced Cancer: Living Each Day

American Cancer Society (1-800-ACS-2345)

Facts on Prostate Cancer (available in Spanish and English)
For Men Only: Prostate Cancer
Sexuality and Cancer for Men

Appendix 4

Sources of Financial Aid for Screening and Treatment

Free or Low-Cost Screening

Many communities have hospitals or private foundations that periodically provide free or low-cost early detection opportunities such as digital rectal exams and PSA blood tests. They are available during a week every September that is designated Prostate Cancer Awareness Week. Call your local cancer treatment center or community hospital for information.

Check with your employer's health office, the social service department of your hospital, or call your local American Cancer Society to find out what's available in your area.

Financial Aid for Hormonal Therapy

Drug manufacturers often provide drugs at low or no cost to people who cannot afford to pay for them. Your urologist or your local American Cancer Society chapter should know about this.

The Schering Corporation of Kenilworth, New Jersey, makers of Eulexin (flutamide), has a program for providing assistance to men needing treatment who cannot afford their drugs. You, your family, or your doctor may apply for benefits for you. The company will need to know the therapy regimen prescribed as well as some financial information from you.

Schering has several plans available depending on whether you have health insurance. The company arranges for you to pick up the drug at your local pharmacy. In addition, Schering provides information and newsletters about prostate cancer treatment.

For information, call 1-800-521-7157 between 9 A.M. and 5 P.M. in all time zones. Your doctor can also write for the *Directory of Prescription Drug Indigent Programs,* which can help locate drugs at low or no cost. It is published by the Pharmaceutical Manufacturers Association in Washington, D.C.

Transportation To and From Treatments

Again, ask your local American Cancer Society chapter or your treatment team about transportation resources. In some communities ACS has a program called *Road to Recovery* designed for this purpose. Trained volunteer drivers take you to treatment and pick you up. There is also a national Corporate Angels program that provides long-distance air transportation to a treatment facility.

See Appendix 1 for information on Cancer Care, which also provides financial aid and transportation to some cancer patients.

Other Sources of Aid

Help for a specific financial problem is usually available somewhere, but it will take some persistent digging and phone calling. Perhaps a family member can help. In addition to the cancer care agencies listed here, other potential sources are community service groups and fraternal and religious organizations in your own neighborhood, public welfare agencies, state and federally funded medical programs such as Medicaid and Medicare.

Appendix 5

What to Know About Medical Insurance

Most Americans now belong to HMOs (health maintenance organizations), which are prepaid health care plans that combine the functions of the insurance company with those of the doctor/hospital by providing health care for a prepaid annual premium. As more and more people enroll, mostly through their employers, more and more problems develop, and the state and federal governments have been introducing legislation to protect patient rights and to outlaw some of the practices that restrict equitable delivery of quality health care.

Most people know very little about their health insurance plans other than the amount of their copayment. Problems relating to confusion about what the plans cover is becoming the norm. It is important that you understand how HMOs affect your treatment options.

HMOs can restrict you to certain doctors and medical centers, diagnostic tests, laboratory pathology procedures, medications, preoperative tests, anesthesia, and home health care. Because these managed care companies deal in volume, they are able to buy services cheaply. For example, they may contract with a particular pathological laboratory so that all of the lab tests of their enrollees are done at that lab. They can buy up enormous amounts of drugs and medications, and this can be good for you, but it may also limit your choice of brand-name drugs.

You need to be well informed about your health plan and call your provider every step along the way if you are unsure of whether or not something is covered. If it is not, there may be some way to get around it. When you are seeking health care, you should always ask a doctor if he or she is prescribing a certain treatment because it is best for you or because it is the only one your health plan will cover.

HMOs generally require you to be treated only through referrals from your primary care physician, known as the gatekeeper. You may be restricted only to the physicians listed in your HMO directory, which means you cannot visit a radiation oncologist or surgeon unless that physician is in the same plan and is referred by the primary care physician. As an example, your primary care physician may refer you to a urologist who is in your plan. The urologist may want to refer you to a radiation therapist who may or may not be in your plan. In some plans, you can go to the radiation therapist on your urologist's referral. But in many, you must go back to your primary care physician and ask for a referral to a radiation therapist. So many complaints have been registered against HMOs for this restriction that some are beginning to change it.

Sometimes HMO restrictions also mean you can seek treatment only in your own neighborhood, city, or state. You may prefer to go to a city where there is a state-of-the-art cancer treatment center.

Another risk is the so-called "gag rule" some managed care plans require of physicians in their network. In order to control costs, as well as the patient's health care, the insurer does not allow the physician to tell a patient about other possible treatment options. Make it a point always to ask a doctor if treatment he or she recommends is the best one for you or is it the only one the insurer will allow.

Many of these restrictions have been challenged and states as well as the federal government have begun passing laws to prevent HMOs from making such decisions. Legislation now prevents bonus sharing arrangements between HMOs and physicians participating in Medicare. When HMOs claimed women having mastectomies could not stay in the hospital overnight, it took an act of Congress to change the law. The rules are changing every day and it is vital to your well-being to keep abreast of the changes in your medical insurance plan.

Here's an example of what to be watchful of if you are in an HMO plan. Let's say you have a transrectal ultrasound needle biopsy of your prostate by a urologist at a comprehensive cancer center. While the doctor's fee is covered, the pathology laboratory costs at that medical center may not be covered because your insurer will pay only for pathology done by a particular outside commercial laboratory, where the insurer has contracted for all pathology work for all members.

However, if you are being treated in a comprehensive cancer center, your urologist will not want to make a surgical decision based on a commercial laboratory biopsy report. He or she will want one done in the same place where the screening was done, where the urologist knows and trusts the quality of the pathology. Physicians generally consider such outside commercial laboratories acceptable for analysis of potassium levels and other minor tests, but many doctors will not trust them for anything as critical as an accurate biopsy interpretation.

Doctors are used to working with other doctors they know as part of a multidisciplinary team to deal with a patient's problems. Comparable training, a common hospital, professional competence, and mutual trust are a part of the "glue" holding together these teams. Trends in health insurance do not necessarily recognize these groups and the teams may be fragmented if one or more physicians necessary to your care is not in your plan. This can put a strain on the doctor-patient relationship if access to what is perceived as necessary or desirable by health care providers is limited by health insurance coverage. If your urologist must get the biopsy slides from another laboratory or hospital and then have them analyzed again, the cost of the biopsy will double and your insurance may not cover it.

Many states have enacted laws to prevent managed care organizations from denying certain kinds of coverage to patients and from making decisions that should be made only by doctors and patients. Here are some of the managed care policies that have been reversed in some states as of the end of 1996.

• A dozen states now guarantee a patient's right to go directly to certain types of specialists without first getting approval from a primary care physician, who insurers consider a gatekeeper. The gatekeeper may severely limit the patient's option in choosing the best and most appropriate care. The new legislation requires health care networks to accept any physician—any willing provider—who has appropriate credentials and agrees to abide by contract terms and conditions. Thus, if you have a doctor who is not in your plan but who is qualified to treat you, the insurance company must pay for the treatment.

• A number of states now require managed care companies and their doctors to tell patients about financial incentives and rules that may affect their care. This requirement applies to Medicare and all other managed care companies.

• At least six states have outlawed gag rules under which some health maintenance organizations threaten to dismiss doctors if they inform patients about alternative care that might add to the costs of treatment. Health care or insurance networks cannot restrict what information practitioners can give patients about care choices.

Before you begin treatment, call your HMO and talk with the patient services department of your medical center. They can often help you get through the red tape and find out exactly what is covered and not covered.

Your Rights to Appeal

You have every right to appeal to your insurance company and renegotiate your coverage. It happens frequently as more and more people become dissatisfied with the restrictions of their health care plans. Some of the HMOs are finding that although their plans work in theory, they do not always work in the real world. Restrictions are beginning to change in some of these plans and they will probably continue to do so until satisfactory health care can be delivered most efficiently. If your health plan will not bend the rules or make an exception in your case, you can appeal to regulatory agencies.

Find out the procedure for appealing a decision by your insurance company. All states are different. In New York you cannot appeal beyond the insurance company, but in California there is an independent board of physicians with no financial stake who will decide on your case.

To file insurance complaints if you think you have been denied coverage or treated unfairly, call your state department of insurance. For managed care providers, call your state department of corporations, division of health care service plans.

Build a Paper Trail

Be sure you get all the coverage and benefits your policy provides. It is a good idea to read your policy and be familiar with it. Keep very careful records of all of your expenses. File claims immediately for covered costs. Many people don't do this and find later that they are confused about what they have claimed and not claimed, what was paid directly to the hospital, and what was reimbursed to them. It is always more difficult to file months later, because in our insurance system the paperwork can become overwhelming.

If you need help in filing claims and understanding how to report your expenses, ask for help. There may be somebody in your family, in the hospital, or at work who is more knowledgeable than you about how health insurance works.

If a claim is turned down, file it again. Call the insurer and be sure to ask for an explanation of why you were turned down. This can happen because of an error in the filing of information from your doctor's office, the hospital, or at the insurance company itself. Claims go through many hands. Always confirm conversations with insurance representatives in writing, or make detailed notes for your file after a telephone conversation.

How to Work Out Your Share of Payments

Medical insurance coverage varies, and even if you are fully covered, you may still have to pay a percentage of the costs for your care. A small copayment percentage on years of hormonal therapy, for example, can be a financial burden. There may also be a limit to your coverage, and after it reaches that limit, you are responsible for the rest of the payment.

Most treatment centers and hospitals have three sets of figures for each patient procedure: what they charge the patient, what the treatment costs them to provide, and what they will receive from medical insurance companies. Therefore, there is some flexibility and you can probably negotiate a fair price in advance on your share of the payment. Find out what all the charges are, how much your insurance will cover, and what remains for you to pay—and how you will pay it. Will you be able to get help from an outside agency? Will the hospital let you pay in installments? Most are willing to arrange a convenient payment plan, although some may demand payment up front, such as the amount of the deductible.

Health Benefits from Employers

Before you leave any job that includes insurance coverage, be sure you are covered by the new job or that you will be able to pick up insurance on your own. You will be covered by your last employer's insurance for 18 months, providing you pay the monthly premiums. This federal law, known as COBRA (Consolidated Omnibus Budget Reconciliation Act), guarantees this coverage.

If a new employer's insurance or your individual insurance will not cover you for a preexisting condition for a year, then keep the COBRA coverage and pay the premiums yourself until your new policy kicks in. You must be able to pay for your follow-up care and surveillance after prostate cancer, which could involve several years.

Health Insurance After Prostate Cancer

For any cancer survivor, health insurance must include the following at the very least: inpatient hospital care, physician services, laboratory and X-ray services, inpatient psychiatric care, outpatient services, and nursing home care. Prescription drug coverage may be important if you will be taking a medication for a long period of time.

The insurer should pay at least 80 percent of the covered services, except possibly for inpatient psychiatric care, which may require that you pay more than 20 percent. Also, the insurer should pay at least $250,000 for catastrophic illness coverage, with you paying no more than 30 percent of your income toward these expenses. Check on the limit. Some policies cover you for up to a million dollars in a lifetime and some have no lifetime cap.

If you are turned down for health insurance coverage because you have had prostate cancer, call your state department of insurance. It may be illegal in your state for an insurance carrier to reject you as long as you are able to pay the premiums. Laws are changing daily as health insurance undergoes changes. Many states are forcing insurers to accept anybody who applies and pays for health insurance, regardless of medical conditions they have been treated for in the past. There are also companies that insure people with high medical risk. These are often the Blue Cross, Blue Shield companies in each state. If you are turned down by a company, find out if the company has an appeals process.

Appendix 6

Your Right to Medical Records

Always keep copies of your medical records. You will want to have them—or at least know what's in them—if you visit other doctors or hospitals. The most useful are your laboratory work studies, staging, scan results, pathology, and operative reports. There are many good reasons for you to possess your medical records. Years from now you will want to have easy access to them if you need them. Your family may need access to your medical information in an emergency. They may not know which doctors or hospitals have your records. Your children and grandchildren may someday need to know your medical history.

Federal law guarantees your right to your medical records. This law is mandated by most states, in spite of opposition from some hospitals and doctors who claim patients will not understand the entries in their records. Your right of privacy is also protected so that others cannot have your medical records without your knowledge and approval. Most hospitals have a medical records department and they sometimes move slowly because a great deal of paper is handled. If you want a copy of any or all of your medical records, you generally have to put the request in writing and complete a form supplied by the hospital. This form legally protects you and the hospital. You should be able to get copies of your records within a few days, however, and sooner if it is urgent. You are entitled to hospital records, doctor records, diagnostic records, X-ray films, pathology slides—all of it.

The best thing to do, as we mentioned throughout the book, is to always get copies of your medical records after each procedure as you progress through treatment. Some physicians have no problem giving you copies. Others tell you to write them a letter requesting copies. They may charge a small processing fee. This is just their way of putting another barrier in the way. It's all a matter of style, because you are entitled to your records. Just keep on insisting.

Appendix 7

Americans with Disabilities Act

Prostate cancer is not a disabling disease, but all cancer survivors are included in the laws protecting the disabled from job discrimination, and rightly so. One in every four cancer survivors experiences some form of job discrimination. If this happens to you, there are laws to protect you and organizations that can help you.

There are more than 8 million cancer survivors in the United States and the number grows daily as cancer treatment becomes more effective and cancer is increasingly cured because of early detection. More than 80 percent of them return to work after treatment. All occupations and professions include cancer survivors, yet many employers still believe the myths that you will not be able to work after you have had cancer, or that you will be taking sick days all too frequently. But most of all, this discrimination is rampant among employers who do not want your medical costs to affect the health insurance premiums they pay for their employees.

In 1992 the Americans with Disabilities Act (ADA) went into effect. This law bans discrimination by employers against qualified workers who have disabilities or histories of disabilities. The law applies to private employers with 15 or more workers. Although we don't consider cancer a disability, some employers obviously do, so it is covered by this law. The Equal Employment Opportunity Commission (EEOC) declared in 1993 that employers cannot refuse to hire people with disabilities and these people must have equal access to health insurance.

Federal employees have been covered since 1973, but private employers were not required to conform to these rules until 1992. The earlier law, the Federal Rehabilitation Act of 1973, also offers protection to employees of the federal government or companies that receive federal funds. This law protects handicapped workers, including cancer survivors, in hiring policies, promotions, transfers, and layoffs. The law includes granting flexible work hours when needed for treatment (such as radiation therapy). Your employer cannot fire you if you are able to do your job.

If you suspect your employer is encouraging you to look for another job or to retire early, or if he or she has used an unfair excuse to fire you, file a complaint with EEOC. This kind of discrimination is often disguised—especially in the age of downsizing—so enforcement is necessary. Unscrupulous employers lay off workers they believe will need more benefits or will often be out sick. One man who had a prostatectomy shortly before he turned 65 was "asked" to retire even though he wanted to continue working. The end of work also meant the end of his benefits at this particular job, yet when he questioned the employer, he was told that a mandatory retirement ruling had just been established. This man was deprived of his benefits as well as a job he had planned to enjoy for several more years. He also had a clear-cut case of discrimination to fight.

Consult the affirmative action officer in your workplace and report your concerns that you are being forced out of your job or treated differently and unfairly. The company cannot retaliate by firing you. Look around for comparisons in your workplace. Did they let another employee return after a heart attack? If they do not reinstate you, you have 180 days to file a complaint with your state human rights commission and 300 days to file with the EEOC. Some attorneys will take on this kind of case without a fee and then get a percentage of the settlement later.

If You Change Jobs

Never discuss your health when you are looking for a new job. You do not need to reveal any information about your prostate cancer treatment or any other medical condition. Employers are not allowed to ask you about your health or to require a preemployment physical exam or health history designed to screen out people with disabilities. Medical questions can be asked only after you are offered the job, and then only if the questions relate specifically to your job. You cannot be asked to reveal anything about prostate cancer if it does not interfere with your ability to work.

Where to Get Help

Many attorneys specialize as advocates and litigators on behalf of people with catastrophic illness. They can help you understand your rights under the Americans with Disabilities Act, as well as your State Human Rights Law, and the Family and Medical Leave Act. There is advice available on how to handle job interviews and what to tell your employer and on what health benefits fall under the Employee Retirement Income Security Act (ERISA). Here are some sources of information:

- EEOC at 1-800-USA-EEOC (1-800-872-3362).
- National Coalition for Cancer Survivorship (NCCS) at 301-585-2616. This organization offers information and sometimes legal referrals.
- Your hospital social workers may also know about laws in your state and the agencies involved in enforcing those laws.
- Your congressional representative or senator.
- The NCI guide, *Facing Forward,* which has work-related information.
- Your local American Cancer Society chapter may be able to provide you with state-specific information about your state and federal law, including the text of the recent Americans with Disabilities law. ACS also has a booklet explaining the Americans with Disabilities Act and your legal rights pertaining to jobs and health insurance. Another helpful publication is *Cancer: Your Job, Insurance, and the Law.*

Appendix 8

Prostate Cancer Clinical Trials

There are many important prostate cancer clinical trials in progress, although not all are available to patients seeking treatment for advanced prostate cancer. For other cancers, there are more often trials of new chemotherapy drugs, but prostate cancer so far lacks an effective treatment with chemotherapy.

The prostate cancer treatment trials, for example, include the participation of men who do not have the disease. Studies to compare the survival rates of men who had surgery with those who did nothing would not afford you access to new or cutting-edge hormonal therapy. The most interesting clinical trials involve intermittent hormonal therapy (see Chapter 13).

Talk with your physician about trials for which you may qualify that might be beneficial for your treatment. Participants in clinical trials are scattered around the United States, usually in comprehensive cancer centers or university teaching hospitals. Study participants have similar prognoses and are part of the same protocol with careful observation and reporting by the physicians. The purpose of the study is to find out how effective a new treatment is, so a number of patients are treated and followed with surveillance for a certain number of years.

Before a drug is used in studies on human patients, it must go through many levels of testing. First it is tested in the laboratory (in vitro), then in animals (in vivo), and finally in controlled studies of human volunteer patients. These are clinical studies. Although most of the drugs used in these trials are already known to be effective, there is not yet enough knowledge to be certain how much and for how long they should be administered for maximum effectiveness. For example, nilutamide, a recently approved antiandrogen similar to flutamide, only came into use in the late 1990s after many years of trials. Each clinical trial tries to answer certain questions in order to find new and better ways to help cancer patients. If, after the designated number of years, a trial shows that a certain standard works better than others, then it may become the new standard treatment.

There may be a clinical trial in progress at the treatment center you choose or one of your physicians may be involved in such a trial. Many doctors participate in these trials, so ask your urologist. Becoming part of the trial means that your progress through the treatment is monitored closely and the data are included and analyzed with data from many other patients. The best trials involve patients not only with a similar prognosis but with other similarities such as age, prostate volume, race, and environmental background.

If you are highly motivated to undergo unproved treatment and are not burdened with additional medical problems, you may be a good candidate for participation in a clinical trial. By joining a clinical trial, you are not becoming a guinea pig. Consider yourself fortunate to have access to the cutting edge of medical treatment, which may be the most effective to date. Like most opportunities in life, there is risk, but if you discuss it thoughtfully with your doctor—and possibly get a second opinion—you should be able to make an informed decision. It is essential that you feel trust and confidence in the care you will get if you participate in a clinical study.

The National Cancer Institute (NCI) has several large-scale studies on prostate cancer that will still be in progress when this book is published.

• The 7-year PCPT (Prostate Cancer Prevention Trial) seeks to determine if finasteride (Proscar) can prevent the disease. Proscar blocks 5-alpha reductase in the prostate and prevents the conversion of testosterone to DHT. The study is enrolling 18,000 men for 7 to 10 years, aged 55 and older, who do not have prostate cancer. Some will receive Proscar and others a placebo. At the end of the study each man will have a biopsy to see if there is a latent cancer in his prostate.

Using the idea that eunuchs, who are castrated as infants, never get prostate cancer, researchers believe there must be a point in the sequence of developmental events when such chemoprevention might work. Prostate cancer has an initiation stage when men who are 50 years of age have a 20 percent chance of having a histologic or latent prostate cancer.

The next stage is the progression phase, which is different in white men, blacks, and Asians. Only 10 percent of Asian men will develop clinical prostate cancer, which is half the rate of white and black men.

• The Prostate Cancer Intervention Versus Observation Trial (PIVOT) is following 2,000 men over a 15-year period. This study hopes to determine whether or not prostatectomy for early prostate cancer is any more effective than watchful waiting. We will not have the results until early in the 21st century.

• The 10-year PLCO (Prostate, Lung, Colorectal, and Ovarian Cancer) Trial is enrolling 148,000 men and women between the ages of 60 and 74 to determine if widespread screening will save lives from these four cancers.

The National Cancer Institute can provide you with the latest information about where clinical trials are taking place and what the qualifications are for participants. Ask for the Community Clinical Oncology Program list of medical centers in the United States selected by NCI to participate in the newest protocols. Call the NCI Cancer Information Hotline at 1-800-4-CANCER.

What to Ask About Clinical Trials

To be part of a controlled study, you will need to give your signed consent to take the treatment in a hospital or clinical setting or in a physician's office with special rigid standards of monitoring and record keeping.

Before you consent to join a clinical trial, you need to know if it is a bonafide and approved trial. Always check with your doctor about the study, the institution, and the drug being tested. Check with the U.S. Food and Drug Administration office nearest you to find out if the study is approved by this agency. Also, ask for the American Cancer Society pamphlet called *Questionable, Alternative, and Complementary Treatments of Cancer: General Information.*

Before you can make up your mind about joining one of these trials, there are many things to know. Most important, you want to know if the physicians running the study are going to provide you with care the same way your own doctor would. Or, will they be simply supervising your treatment? You need to know who to call when you have a problem or a question, whether or not you can drop out, and if the trial is approved by the FDA, the NCI, or other official organizations.

Experimental or investigational treatments are often not covered by medical insurance; however, this tends to be decided on an individual basis depending on the particular study and your particular insurance carrier.

Appendix 9

Glossary

5-Alpha reductase. An enzyme that converts testosterone to dihydrotestosterone (DHT), which is its more potent metabolite.

ACTH. Adrenocorticotropic hormone, which causes adrenal glands to produce androgens.

Adenocarcinoma. Cancer that appears in glandular tissue such as the prostate.

Adjuvant therapy. Treatment given in addition to the primary therapy.

Adrenal androgen. A male hormone produced by the adrenal glands; adrenal androgens account for about 5 percent of the body's androgens.

Aminoglutethimide. A drug used for hormone-refractory prostate cancer to suppress production of androgens by the adrenal glands.

Anastomosis. The juncture where two organs are surgically joined, such as where the bladder and urethra are joined after removal of the prostate.

Androgen. Male hormone such as testosterone.

Androgen blockade. Use of drugs to interrupt the activity of male hormones.

Antiandrogen. A drug used to block the activity of male hormones.

Benign. A growth that is not cancer.

Benign prostatic hyperplasia (BPH). Enlargement of the prostate; noncancerous.

Bicalutamide. Casodex, an antiandrogen.

Biofeedback. A method of self-monitoring and controlling some bodily systems. Used to reduce muscle tension, blood pressure, nausea, stress, and pain.

215

Biopsy. Removal of tissue for histologic analysis, microscopic study, or pathologic evaluation.

Bladder neck. Thickened muscle where the bladder joins the urethra. On signal from the brain, this muscle can either tighten or relax to control flow of urine from the bladder to the urethra.

Bladder neck contracture. A complication of surgery that causes scarring of the tissue and possible urinary problems. Could require additional surgery to correct.

Brachytherapy. Interstitial radiation treatment; the placement of radioactive seeds into the prostate.

Carcinoma. Cancer that begins in the lining or covering tissues of an organ (epithelium) such as the prostate.

Cardura. Doxazosin, a medication used for BPH to relax the prostate muscle.

Castration. The removal of male hormones either through surgical removal of the testicles or with drugs that inhibit hormone production.

Chemotherapy. Systemic cancer treatment with medications that reach every cell in the body.

Clinical biopsy. Pathological study of prostate tissue taken with a needle to determine the presence or absence of cancer cells.

Clinical trials. Controlled research studies of cancer treatments on a fixed number of patients–volunteers–designed to answer certain questions and determine better ways to prevent, detect, or treat cancer.

CT scan. Also CAT. Computerized axial tomography. A cross-sectional X-ray used in diagnosis and radiation treatment planning.

Cystitis. Infection and inflammation of the bladder, which is a possible short-lived side effect of radiation therapy. Causes painful urination.

DES. Diethylstilbestrol, a synthetic estrogen, used in treatment of prostate cancer.

DHT. Dihydrotestosterone. A more potent metabolized form of testosterone.

Differentiated. The resemblance of cancer cells to normal cells. Well-differentiated tumor cells closely resemble normal cells and are, therefore, believed to be less aggressive.

Digital rectal exam (DRE). The doctor inserts a lubricated, gloved finger into the rectum and feels for abnormalities of the prostate, anus, or rectum.

Diploid. Cell population that contains the normal amount of DNA material.

DNA. Deoxyribonucleic acid. Material in the nucleus (brain of the cell) that codes what that cell will become.

Dysplasia. Abnormal growth of cells.

Dysuria. Burning sensation when urinating.

Epidural. Anesthesia. Medication delivered to the spinal nerve area that causes analgesia from the waist down.

Estrogen. A female sex hormone.

External beam radiation. Radiation treatment that is delivered from outside the body.

Flutamide. Eulexin, an antiandrogen used in hormonal treatment.

Frozen section. A small piece of a larger piece of tissue taken out during a biopsy that is flash frozen for instant analysis by a pathologist using a microscope to determine whether cancer is present.

FSH. Follicle-stimulating hormone produced by the pituitary gland to activate sperm-forming tubules in the testicles.

Genetic markers. Abnormalities found in the genes that indicate the presence of cancer or the potential to develop into cancer.

Glans. Head of the penis.

Goserelin. Zoladex, a synthetic LHRH agonist/antagonist used in hormonal treatment.

Gray. A unit of measure for radiation treatment. Abbreviated as Gy.

Gy. *See* **Gray.**

Hematuria. Blood in the urine.

Histologic diagnosis. Study of what's under the microscope, the most minute branch of anatomic study. The information in your pathology report.

Hormone refractory. Cancer cells that are no longer responsive to hormonal treatment.

Hormone therapy. Treatment for prostate cancer that interferes with the body's production of male hormones.

Hyperplasia. Abnormal growth of cells due to rapid cell multiplication.

Hytrin. Terazocin, a muscle relaxant used to treat BPH.

Impotence. The inability for a man to achieve an erection. Also called erectile dysfunction.

Incontinence. Involuntary loss of urine.

Internal radiation therapy. Treatment from radioactive seeds implanted in the tumor, also known as interstitial radiation.

Invasive. Cancer that can or has spread from its original site.

Irradiation. Radiation therapy.

Ketoconazole. An antifungal agent used to inhibit production of androgens in hormone-refractory cancer.

Lesion. A tumor, mass, or other abnormality.

Leuprolide. Lupron, an LHRH agonist/antagonist used in hormonal treatment.

Local anesthesia. A drug that numbs only an area of your body but allows you to remain awake.

Luteinizing hormone (LH). This hormone is secreted by the pituitary gland. It stimulates secretion of androgen by the testicles.

Luteinizing hormone-releasing hormone (LHRH). This hormone is secreted by the brain to stimulate the secretion of LH by the pituitary gland.

Lymph. The almost colorless fluid that bathes body tissues and carries cells that help fight infection. Operates much like the circulatory system.

Lymphatic system. The tissues and organs, including the bone marrow, spleen, thymus, and lymph nodes, that produce and store cells that fight infection and disease.

Lymphedema. Swelling, usually of the lower extremities due to obstruction of the lymphatic system.

Lymph nodes. Small, bean-shaped organs located along the lymphatic system. Nodes filter bacteria or cancer cells that may travel through the lymphatic system. Also called lymph glands.

MAB. Maximal androgen blockade. Hormonal therapy using drugs to completely block the production and activity of male hormones.

Magnetic resonance imaging (MRI). Radiological study that utilizes a magnet to generate cross-sectional images of the body. Gives excellent detail about soft tissue densities. Used to detect bone cancer and other conditions, and to sometimes evaluate lymph nodes.

Malignant. Cancerous.

Mass. A lesion, tumor, lump, or nodule.

Metastasis. The spread of cancer from one part of the body to another.

Metastatic disease. Cancer that has spread from its original site to other parts of the body, most commonly the bone, lung, liver, brain, and lymph nodes.

Metastatic lesions. A cancerous lesion or tumor at another site that has the same cancer cells as the original tumor.

Negative margins. *See* **Surgical margins.**

Negative nodes. Lymph nodes showing no signs of prostate cancer.

Neoplasia. Proliferation of cells whose growth exceeds and is uncoordinated with other cells. *See* **PIN.**

Nilutamide. Nilandron, an antiandrogen used in hormonal treatment.

Nocturia. The need to get up frequently at night to urinate.

Noninvasive. In situ cancer that does not spread outside the prostate lining.

Occult cancer. Cancer that is hidden from view, not detectable by clinical methods alone.

Oncologist. A doctor who specializes in treating cancer. Medical oncologist, urologic surgeon, radiation oncologist, etc.

Orchiectomy. The surgical removal of the testicles (testes).

Palliative. Treatment that relieves symptoms such as pain but does not cure.

Pathologic diagnosis. A histologic diagnosis (biopsy) report on the state of the microscopic particles of the tumor. The final report after full pathologic evaluation.

Pathologist. A doctor who identifies diseases by studying cells and tissues under a microscope.

Perineal prostatectomy. Surgical removal of the prostate through an incision in the area between the scrotum and the anus.

PIN. Prostatic intraepithelial neoplasia. Believed by some pathologists to be a premalignant lesion if it is high grade.

Pituitary gland. Located at the base of the brain, this gland produces a variety of hormones to stimulate the testicles and other glands to release hormones.

Positive lymph nodes. Lymph nodes that contain cancer cells.

Positive margins. *See* **Surgical margins.**

Premalignant. A condition that indicates a significant potential for becoming cancer.

Proctitis. Irritation and pain in the rectum and anus, causing diarrhea and bleeding, a potential side effect of radiation therapy.

Prognostic indicators. All elements of the disease used to determine prognosis and treatment, such as size and location of the tumor and behavior of the cells involved, number of nodes, patient's age, etc.

Prostatectomy. Surgical removal of the prostate.

PSA. Prostate-specific antigen. An enzyme in the semen of every man with a prostate that can become elevated in the blood of men who have prostate cancer or BPH (benign prostatic hyperplasia). Functions to liquefy the seminal fluid.

RAD. A unit of measure for radiation treatment. 100 rads is equivalent to 1 Gy.

Radiation oncologist. A physician who specializes in radiation treatment.

Radiation therapy. Treatment with high-energy rays from X-rays or other sources to kill or slow cancer cells. Also reduces pain from cancer spread to bone by killing tumor at this site.

Rectum. The lower part of the large intestine (colon) that ends in the anal opening.

Resectoscope. Fiberoptic instrument used to remove prostate tissue through the penile urethra with an electrical cautery loop.

Retropubic prostatectomy. Surgical removal of the prostate through an open incision in the lower abdomen.

Semen. The fluid produced by the prostate, seminal vesicles, and other glands of the male reproductive system to carry sperm through the urethra and penis during ejaculation.

Seminal vesicles. Two glands, like small bunches of grapes, at the top of the prostate and behind the bladder, which produce the sticky substance in semen.

Sphincter. Muscle that can tighten or relax to close or open a body passage or opening, such as the bladder or rectum. The internal sphincter is located at the bladder neck. The external sphincter is in the pelvic floor muscle.

Staging. The process of learning whether cancer has spread from its original site to another part of the body. Clinical staging is based on history and physical examination. Pathologic staging is based on findings after surgery.

Surgical margins. Cut edges at the apex and base of the prostate specimen removed during surgery and studied by a pathologist to check for the presence of tumor cells. If no cancer has reached the edge of the tissue, margins are negative. If cancer has reached the edge, margins are positive.

Testicles. Two egg-shaped glands that produce sperm and testosterone, located below the penis in the pouchlike scrotum.

Testosterone. A male hormone produced primarily in the testicles.

Transurethral resection of the prostate (TURP). An endoscopic instrument is inserted through the penis to remove noncancerous prostate tissue.

TRUS. *See* **Ultrasound.**

Tumor. A mass of tissue, lesion, lump, or nodule.

Ultrasound. A diagnostic test that bounces sound waves off tissues and converts the echoes into pictures. Transrectal ultrasound uses a probe inserted into the rectum to evaluate the prostate.

Urethral stricture. A complication of surgery resulting in scarring of tissue in the urethra and narrowing of the channel that carries urine and semen through the urethra. Requires corrective surgery.

Urologist. A physician who specializes in the treatment of the diseases of the male sexual and urinary tract, and the urinary tract in women.

Vas deferens. Tube through which sperm travels from each testicle to the ejaculatory duct of the urethra.

Index

Absorbent pads, for incontinence, 166
ACTH (adrenocorticotropic hormone), 8
Activity, after surgery, 95–96
Advance directives, surgery and, 86
Advanced prostate cancer, treatment for,
    119–131
  hormonal therapy; *See* Hormonal
    therapy
Age/Aging
  as prostate cancer risk factor, 29
  PSA adjustment for, 50–51
American Association of Sex Educators,
    Counselors and Therapists
    (AASECT), 192
American Cancer Society, 188, 198
American College of Surgeons Commit-
    tee on Cancer, 190
Americans with Disabilities Act, 208–210
American Urological Association, 191
Anesthesiologists, 92
Antiandrogens, 126–127
Antioxidants, 35
Appeal, rights to, health/medical
    insurance, 204
Artificial sphincter, for incontinence, 167

Banking your own blood, for surgery, 88
Bibliography, 197
Biofeedback
  for incontinence, 165
  treatment aids, 147–148
Bone scan, 43–44
Bowel problems, from radiation therapy,
    105
BPH (benign prostatic hyperplasia), 6, 8,
    9–22, 26
  diagnosis of, 14–15
  dynamic and static prostate, 12–13
  medications for, 16–17

microwave treatment for, 19–20
Proscar (finesteride) for, 12, 16–17
prostate cancer and, 36
PSA (prostate-specific antigen) and, 12
surgical treatment of, 17–18
symptoms of, 13–14
treatment of, 15–18
Brachytherapy (interstitial radiation),
    111–118
  candidates for, 113–114
  complications of, 115–116
  procedure, 112–115
  questions to ask, 117–118
  rectal problems, 116
  sexual concerns, 116–117
  side effects, short-term, of implants,
    116–117
  treatment planning, 114
  treatment team, 114–115
  urinary complications, 116
BRCA1, 30

Cancer; *See* Prostate cancer
Cancer Care, 189–190
CancerFax, 187
CancerNet, 188
Candidates, for brachytherapy, 113–114
CaP Cure, 191
Catheters
  after surgery, 96
  functioning with, 163–164
CAT scan, 26
Cell immunity to treatment, hormonal
    therapy and, 123–124
Central zone, 7
Checklists
  for going home after surgery, 97–98
  pre-surgery, 89–90
Circulating androgens, 129

Clinical biopsy
  as diagnostic test, 41, 47
  grading and staging report, 57–58
COBRA, 206
Collagen implants, for incontinence,
      166–167
Combination therapies, radiation
      therapy, 106–107
Complications, of brachytherapy,
      115–116
Computerized axial tomography (CAT)
      scan, 44
Consenting, to surgery, 85–86
Controversy, of watchful waiting, 64–65
Corticosteroids, hormonal therapy
      and, 130
Costs
  of hormonal therapy, 131
  of radiation therapy, 109–110
  of screening, diagnostic, 45–46
  of treatment
      restoring potency, 177
      treatment decisions and, 157

Decision, on treatment; See Treatment
Degrees of difference in early cancer,
      watchful waiting and, 65–67
Density, PSA adjustment for, 51
Depression, postoperative, 96–97
Development, of prostate cancer, 23–27
DHT (dihydrotestosterone), 8, 11
Diagnosis, of BPH, 14–15
Diagnostic tests, 39–48
  bone scan, 43–44
  clinical biopsy, 41, 47
      grading and staging, 57–58
  computerized axial tomography (CAT)
      scan, 44
  costs of screening, 45–46
  digital rectal exam (DRE), 39–41
  magnetic resonance imaging (MRI),
      44–45
  performance of, 47
  ProstaScint scan, 45
  screening
      costs of, 45–46

questions about, 46–47
side effects of, 47
staging tests, other, 43
transrectal ultrasound (TRUS), 41–43
transurethral resection of the prostate
      (TURP), 43
urologist's role in, 46
Diet
  health and, 182–184
  modification of, for incontinence,
      165–166
  as prostate cancer risk factor, 31–35
Differentiation, of cells, 23
Digital rectal exam (DRE), 39–41
Diseases of the prostate, 9–22
  BPH; See BPH (benign prostatic
      hyperplasia)
  PIN (prostatic intraepithelial neopla-
      sia), 21–22
  prostatitis, 20–21
DNA, 23
Doubling time, 24
Downstaging, 57
DRE (direct rectal exam), 10, 15, 20, 25
Drinking fluids, after surgery, 96
Dynamic and static prostate, BPH and,
      12–13

Early localized prostate cancer, 61–118
  brachytherapy; See Brachytherapy
      (interstitial radiation)
  external beam radiation therapy; See
      External beam radiation therapy
  surgery: radical prostatectomy; See
      Radical prostatectomy
  watchful waiting, 63–67
      controversy of, 64–65
      degrees of difference in early
      cancer, 65–67
Early treatment, watchful waiting and,
      64–65
Eastern techniques, treatment aids,
      148–149
Eating and drinking, after surgery, 96
Emotional responses, treatment decisions
      and, 154–155

Enema, self-administered, surgery and, 90–91

Environment, as prostate cancer risk factor, 31–32

Erectile Dysfunction Unit, 193

Erections, mechanics of, 170

ERISA, 210

Estrogen, hormonal therapy and, 125–126

Exercise, after surgery, 95–96

External beam radiation therapy, 99–110
  bowel problems from, 105
  combination therapies, 106–107
  cost of, 109–110
  follow-up care, 107–108
  how it works, 101–104
  long-term side effects, 105–106
  neoadjuvant hormone therapy, 106
  radiation oncologists, 108–109
  radiation treatment team, 108–109
  "salvage" surgery and, 107
  short-term side effects, 104–105
  side effects
    long-term, 105–106
    short-term, 104–105
  simulation: planning treatment, 102–103
  skin irritation from, 104
  technicians, 109
  three-dimensional (3D) conformal technique, 101–102
  treatment process, 103–104
  urinary changes from, 104–105

External condoms, for incontinence, 166

External sphincters, strengthening, 164–165

Family
  history, as prostate cancer risk factor, 29–30
  sharing treatment decision making, 155–156

Fasting, preoperative, 90

Fat consumption, reducing, 183

Financial aid, 199–200

Finesteride; See Proscar (finesteride)

Follow-up care, radiation therapy, 107–108

Free publications, 197–198

FSH (follicle-stimulating hormone), 8

Genes, prostate cancer, 29

Geography, of the prostate, 7

Gleason score, 54–55

Global incontinence, 162

Glossary, 215–222

Going home, after surgery, checklist for, 97–98

Grading and staging, 54–59
  clinical biopsy report, 57–58
  downstaging, 57
  Gleason score, 54–55
  health insurance and biopsy, 58
  second pathology opinion, 59
  staging, 56–57
  tests, other, 43
  TNM system, 55–56
  upstaging, 57

Growth and development, of the prostate, 3

Health, monitoring, 178–185
  diet and, 182–184
  exercising and, 183–184
  fat consumption, reducing, 183
  PSA surveillance, 178–182

Health/Medical insurance, 201–206
  after prostate cancer, 206
  appeal, rights to, 204
  biopsy and, 58
  employers, health benefits from, 205–206
  paper trails and, 204–205
  surgery and, 86–87

High-animal fat diet, as prostate cancer risk factor, 32–34

HMOs; See also Health/Medical insurance
  treatment centers and, 140–141

Home Delivery Incontinent, 191

Home health care, surgery and, 85

Hormonal therapy, 121–131
  antiandrogens, 126–127
  cell immunity to treatment, 123–124

Hormonal therapy *(continued)*
  circulating androgens, reducing, 129
  corticosteroids, 130
  cost of, 131
  estrogen, 125–126
  financial aid for, 199–200
  hormone-refractory cancer, 128–131
  ketoconazole, 130
  LHRH agonists-antagonists, 126
  maximal androgen blockade (MAB),
    127–128
  orchiectomy, 124
  secondary orchiectomy, 129
  synthetic hormones, 124–125
Hormone-refractory cancer, 27, 128–131
Hormones, role of, 7–8
Hospital support staff, surgery and,
  84–85
HPC1 (hereditary prostate cancer), 29
Hyperplasia, 10
  benign prostatic; *See* BPH (benign
    prostatic hyperplasia)

Impotence; *See also* Potency, restoring
  information resources, 192–193
  radical prostatectomy and, 74–75
Impotence Anonymous, 192
Impotence Information Center, 192
Impotence Institute of America, 193
Incisions, caring for, after surgery,
  94–95
Incontinence
  coping with, 161–167
    absorbent pads, 166
    artificial sphincter, 167
    biofeedback and, 165
    catheters, 163–164
    collagen implants, 166–167
    diet modification and, 165–166
    external condoms, 166
    external sphincters, 164–165
    global incontinence, 162
    kegels and, 164–165
    overflow incontinence, 162
    protective products, 166
    severe incontinence, 166–167

    stress incontinence, 162
    urge incontinence, 162
  information resources, 191
  radical prostatectomy and, 74
Information resources, 187–193
  impotence, 192–193
  incontinence, 191
In situ cancer, 24
Interstitial radiation; *See* Brachytherapy
  (interstitial radiation)
Invasive cancer, 24
IVP (intravenous pyelogram), 15

Kegels, 164–165
Ketoconazole
  aminoglutethimide, 130–131
  hormonal therapy and, 130

Laparoscopic technique, radical
  prostatectomy, 76
Laser therapy; *See* VLAP (visual laser
  ablation of the prostate)
LH (luteinizing hormone), 8, 11
LHRH (luteinizing hormone-releasing
  hormone), 8, 11, 16
  agonists-antagonists, 126
Long-term side effects, radiation
  therapy, 105–106
Lymphadenectomy, radical
  prostatectomy and, 75–76

Magnetic resonance imaging (MRI),
  44–45
Male reproductive tract, 4
Margins, positive, radical prostatectomy
  and, 78–79
Maximal androgen blockade (MAB),
  127–128
Mechanics, of the prostate, 5–6
Medicaid, 142
Medical insurance; *See* Health/Medical
  insurance
Medical opinions, additional, treatment
  decisions and, 152–153
Medical records, rights to, 207
Medicare, 142

Medications
  for BPH, 16–17
  reviewing, for surgery, 87–88
Meditation, treatment aids, 148
Metastatic cancer, 25–26
Microwave treatment, for BPH, 19–20

National Association for Continence
    (NAFC), 191
National Cancer Institute (NCI), 16, 187,
    197–198
National Coalition for Cancer Survivor-
    ship (NCCS), 190
National Kidney and Urologic Diseases
    Information Clearinghouse, 191
NCI Cancer Information Service
    Hotline, 187
Neoadjuvant hormone therapy, 106
Nerve-sparing technique, radical
    prostatectomy, 70–71
Neurovascular bundles, 5
Nonmedical aids, to treatment; See
    Treatment
Not for Men Only, 193

Oncologists, radiation, 108–109
Oncology, psychiatric, 139–140
Operating rooms, 92–93
Orchiectomy, 124
Other doctors, alerting, surgery and,
    83–84
Overflow incontinence, 162

Pain, after surgery, controlling, 93–94
Paper trails, health/medical insurance
    and, 204–205
Pathology
  of the prostate specimen, 76–77
  report, 77–78
  second opinion, grading and staging,
    59
Paying for treatment, 140
Penile prostheses, 176
Perineal approach, radical prostatectomy,
    71–72
Peripheral zone, 7

Pharmacologic erection program (PEP),
    174–176
Physicians
  choosing, 135–142
    psychiatric oncology, 139–140
    urologists, 135–136
  Medicare and Medicaid, 142
PIN (prostatic intraepithelial neoplasia),
    21–22, 29
Potency, restoring, 168–178, 192
  cost of treatment, 177
  erections, mechanics of, 170
  penile prostheses, 176
  pharmacologic erection program
    (PEP), 174–176
  transurethral therapy, 172–174
  treatment options, 170–171
  vacuum erection device (VED), 171–172
Potency Restored, 192
Preoperative fasting, 90
Preoperative tests, 89
Private counseling, treatment aids, 146–
    147
Proscar (finesteride), 12
  for BPH, 16–17
ProstaScint scan, 45
Prostate
  diseases of; See Diseases of the prostate
  geography of, 7
  growth and development, 3
  hormones, role of, 7–8
  mechanics of, 5–6
  primer on, 3–8
Prostate cancer, 8
  advanced, treatment for, 119–131
  clinical trials, 211–214
  development of, 23–27
  early localized; See Early localized
    prostate cancer
  hormone-refractory, 27
  metastatic, 25–26; See also Hormonal
    therapy
  PIN (prostatic intraepithelial neopla-
    sia) and, 21–22
  risk factors; See Risks/Risk factors
  symptoms of, 24–25

Prostate Health Council, The, 190–191
Prostatitis, 20–21
Prostatron, 19–20
Prostheses, penile, 176
Protective products, for incontinence, 166
Proximity, to treatment centers, 156–157
PSA (prostate-specific antigen), 6, 16–17, 20, 21, 23, 30–31
    age, adjustment for, 50–51
    BPH and, 12
    as controversial test, 48–53
    density, adjustment for, 51
    measurement of, 49
    monitoring, 178–182
    race, adjustment for, 50–51
    screening dilemmas, 52–53
    velocity, adjustment for, 51
Psychiatric oncology, 139–140

Questions to ask
    brachytherapy, 117–118
    radical prostatectomy, 79–81

Race
    as prostate cancer risk factor, 30–31
    PSA adjustment for, 50–51
Radiation oncologists, 108–109
Radiation therapy
    brachytherapy; See Brachytherapy (interstitial radiation)
    external beam; See External beam radiation therapy
    treatment team, 108–109
Radical prostatectomy, 68–81
    impotence and, 74–75
    for incontinence, 74
    laparoscopic technique, 76
    lymphadenectomy and, 75–76
    margins, positive, 78–79
    nerve-sparing technique, 70–71
    pathology
        of the prostate specimen, 76–77
        report, 77–78
    perineal approach, 71–72

questions to ask about surgery, 79–81
recurrence risks, 79
retropubic approach, 70
risks of, 73–75
shrinking tumor before, 72–73
technique of, 69–70
traditional lymphadenectomy, 75–76
Recovery, 159–185
    health, monitoring; See Health, monitoring
    for incontinence; See Incontinence
    potency; See Potency, restoring
Recovery of Male Potency (ROMP), 193
Rectal problems, brachytherapy, 116
Recurrence risks, radical prostatectomy and, 79
Reproductive tract, male, 4
Retropubic approach, 70
Risks/Risk factors, 28–36
    aging, 29
    antioxidants and, 35
    BPH, 35–36
    diet, 31–35
    environment, 31–32
    family history, 29–30
    fruits/vegetables and, 34–35
    high-animal fat diet, 32–34
    race, 30–31
    of radical prostatectomy, 73–75
    soy and, 35
    sunbelt theory, 35–36
    tomatoes and, 34–35
    unproven, 35–36
    vasectomy, 36

"Salvage" surgery, 107
Screening
    costs of, 45–46
    dilemmas, PSA and, 52–53
Secondary orchiectomy, 129
Second pathology opinion, 59
Selected studies, 194–196
Seminal fluid, 6–7
Sex Information and Education Council of the U.S. (SIECUS), 192

Sexual concerns, brachytherapy, 116–117
Short-term side effects
  of implants, 116–117
  radiation therapy, 104–105
Shrinking tumors, before radical
        prostatectomy, 72–73
Side effects
  of diagnostic tests, 47
  long-term, radiation therapy, 105–106
  Proscar (finesteride), 16–17
  short-term, radiation therapy, 104–105
Simulation: planning treatment, radiation
        therapy, 102–103
Skin irritation, from radiation therapy,
        104
Soy, 35
Sperm, 6–7
Sphincters, artificial, for incontinence,
        167
Staging; See Grading and staging
Stress incontinence, 162
Stress reduction, treatment aids, 147–149
Stroma, 4
Studies, selected, 194–196
Support groups, 145–146
Support services, at treatment centers,
        138–139
Surgery
  advance directive, 86
  after, 93–97
    activity and exercise, 95–96
    catheters, 96
    depression, 96–97
    eating and drinking, 96
    incisions, caring for, 94–95
    pain, controlling, 93–94
  anesthesiologist, meeting with, 92
  banking your own blood, 88
  for BPH, 17–18
  checklist, 89–90
  consenting to, 85–86
  day and night before, 90–91
  day of, 91–93
  enema, self-administered, 90–91
  going home, checklist for, 97–98

health insurance considerations, 86–87
home health care, 85
hospital support staff, 84–85
medications, reviewing, 87–88
in the operating room, 92–93
other doctors, alerting, 83–84
packing for, 91
preoperative fasting, 90
preoperative tests, 89
radical prostatectomy; See Radical
        prostatectomy
treatment team, meeting, 83
the weeks before, 82–83
Symptoms
  of BPH, 13–14
  of prostate cancer, 24–25
    metastatic, 26
  of prostatitis, 20
Synthetic hormones, 124–125

Technicians, radiation therapy, 109
Three-dimensional (3D) conformal
        technique, 101–102
TNM system, 55–56
Tomatoes, 34–35
Traditional lymphadenectomy, 75–76
Transition zone, 7
Transportation, financial aid for, 199–200
Transrectal ultrasound (TRUS), 41–43
Transurethral therapy, 172–174
  resection of the prostate (TURP), 43
Treatment
  for advanced prostate cancer, 119–131
  of BPH, 15–18
  centers
    choosing, 135–142
    comprehensive, 137–138
    support services at, 138–139
    HMOs, 140–141
    Medicare and Medicaid, 142
    paying for treatment, 140
    proximity to, 156–157
  decision on, 150–157
    cost of treatment and, 157
    emotional responses, 154–155

Treatment *(continued)*
    medical conditions, other, 154
    medical opinions, additional,
        152–153
    proximity to treatment centers,
        156–157
    shared with family, 155–156
for early localized prostate cancer; *See*
        Early localized prostate cancer
nonmedical aids to, 143–149
    biofeedback, 147–148
    eastern techniques, 148–149
    meditation, 148
    private counseling, 146–147
    stress reduction, 147–149
    support from family and friends, 144
    support groups, 145–146
    visualization, 148
    in the workplace, 144–145
planning of, brachytherapy, 114
potency, restoring, 170–171
process, radiation therapy, 103–104
of prostatitis, 20–21
team
    brachytherapy, 114–115
    meeting with, before surgery, 83
    radiation therapy, 108–109
transportation to, financial aid for, 200

TURP (transurethral resection of the
        prostate), 6, 12, 17–19

Upstaging, 57
Urge incontinence, 162
Urinary changes, from radiation therapy,
        104–105
Urinary complications, brachytherapy,
        116
Urologist's role, in diagnostic tests, 46
Us Too! International, Inc., 189

Vacuum erection device (VED), 171–172
Vas deferens, 5
Vasectomy, 36
Vegetables and fruit, 34–35
Velocity, PSA adjustment for, 51
Visualization, treatment aids, 148
VLAP (visual laser ablation of the
        prostate), 19

Watchful waiting, for early localized
        prostate cancer, 63–67
    controversy of, 64–65
    degrees of difference in early cancer,
        65–67
Workplace, support in, 144–145

The Authors

Marcus H. Loo, M.D., is a clinical assistant professor of urology at Cornell University Medical College in New York City. He obtained his undergraduate engineering and medical degrees from Cornell University. His postgraduate residency training in surgery and urology were at the New York Hospital–Cornell Medical Center. One of his research interests is interracial differences in the incidence of prostate cancer. He is currently president of the Chinese American Medical Society.

Marian Betancourt has been a professional writer and editor for more than 20 years. Her work has appeared in national magazines and newspapers. Since 1990 she has written extensively about medical issues. She is the co-author of *What to Do if You Get Breast Cancer* (Little, Brown 1995), *What to Do if You Get Colon Cancer* (Wiley, 1997), and *Chronic Illness and the Family: A Guide to Living Every Day* (Adams, 1996). She is also the author of *What to Do When Love Turns Violent: A Practical Resource for Women in Abusive Relationships,* published by HarperCollins (1997). She is currently working on a book about women's health for Avon. Betancourt is on the board of the American Society of Journalists and Authors, and is a member of the Author's Guild and the Authors Registry. She lives in Brooklyn.